The Assessment of Sexual and Marital Function

Special Issue of the JOURNAL OF SEX & MARITAL THERAPY

Edited by

Raul C. Schiavi, M.D.

HUMAN SCIENCES PRESS
72 Fifth Avenue   3 Henrietta Street
NEW YORK, NY 10011 ● LONDON, WC2E 8LU

Library of Congress Catalog Number: 79-67275
ISBN:0-87705-468-1
Copyright 1979 by Human Sciences Press

HUMAN SCIENCES PRESS
72 Fifth Avenue
New York, New York 10011

Printed in the United States of America

Volume 5, Number 3   Fall 1979

Journal of Sex & Marital Therapy

AUDIO/VISUAL REVIEWS
Oliver J. W. Bjorksten, MD, Editor

The JOURNAL OF SEX & MARITAL THERAPY provides an active and contemporary forum for the new clinical techniques and conceptualizations that are emerging from the practice of sex and marital therapy. As a clinical and therapeutically oriented journal, it will emphasize information on new therapeutic techniques, research on outcome, special clinical problems, as well as the theoretical parameters of sexual functioning and marital relationships.

MANUSCRIPTS should be submitted to the Editors, *Journal of Sex & Marital Therapy*, 65 East 76th Street, Suite 1A, New York, N.Y. 10021, in triplicate with a 100-word abstract. Sufficient postage should be included to insure return of a manuscript. The entire manuscript, including references, quotations, and tables, should be double-spaced. Style should conform to that found in these pages. References should be numbered in the text in order of citation and should be listed following the style used by INDEX MEDICUS. Footnotes, except for an introductory footnote on the first page, are discouraged. Further information concerning the preparation of manuscripts can be obtained for the editors.

SUBSCRIPTIONS are on an academic year basis: $40 per volume for institutions and $16 for individuals (individual price valid only if paid by personal check and specified for personal use.)

OVERSEAS SUBSCRIPTIONS: Human Sciences Press, 3 Henrietta Street, London WC2E 8LU, England.

ADVERTISING inquiries should be made to the Business Office. BUSINESS OFFICE: Human Sciences Press, 72 Fifth Avenue, New York, N.Y. 10011. (212) 243-6000.

INDEXED in Psychological Abstracts, Excerpta Medica, Social Sciences Citation Index, Current Contents/Social and Behavioral Sciences, Automatic Subject Citation Alert, Current Index to Journals in Education, Community Mental Health Review, Current Literature—Journal of Homosexuality, Human Sexuality Update, Marriage and Family Review, Sociological Abstracts, Public Health Reviews. LISTED in Selected List of Tables of Contents of Psychiatric Periodicals.

Journal of Sex & Marital Therapy
Vol. 5, No. 3, Fall 1979

Editorial

The Assessment of Sexual and Marital Function

The scientific understanding of human behavior depends upon the identification and description of relevant psychological variables and the development of methods of measurement to gather, quantify, and analyze information from individuals and groups. These data provide a basis for judgments about the characteristics of a particular individual or population and for the generation of predictions about future behavior. During the past forty years the field of psychological measurement has been growing at an exponential rate and efforts at the objective assessment of psychological function have resulted in the availability of increasingly sophisticated and precise instruments. The scope of measurement has expanded from its original emphasis on intelligence to include dimensions of human behavior such as attitudes, special abilities, maturation, achievement, and personality. Although the initial attempts at measuring marital adjustment dates back to the 20's, it was not until the beginning of the 60's that serious psychometric efforts concerned with human sexual function were initiated.

In the fall of 1976 this Journal published an issue designed to emphasize the relevance of psychophysiological and endocrine methods for the study of normal and pathological sexual behavior. At the time it was stated that there was "a parallel need for subjective measures of sexual attitudes, arousal and responsiveness and their application together with other psychological dimensions in future psychophysiological investigations." The present issue is devoted in its entirety to the psychological assessment and measurement of sexual and marital functioning.

The first article by Schiavi, Derogatis, Kuriansky, O'Connor and Sharpe provides, after a brief historical and psychometric presentation, a panoramic view of available instruments for the assessment of sexual function and marital interaction. This article originated from the activities of the Research Committee of the Eastern Association for Sex Therapy in response to the need of members of this organization for standardized and objective techniques that could permit the characterization of patient groups, the study of therapeutic process and outcome evaluation of various treatment methods. The list of instruments included in this article, together with their most relevant psychometric characteristics, although not complete, is representative of a range of tests, questionnaires, inventories and scales for the assessment of sexual and marital function.

0092–623X/79/1500–0167$00.95

Nowinski and LoPiccolo emphasize in their article that the use of psychological tests not only have research value but can also contribute significantly to clinical practice. The authors describe the assessment procedures conducted at the Sex Therapy Center of the Department of Psychiatry at Stony Brook and illustrate the central role that a battery of paper and pencil self-report inventories can have in the evaluation and treatment of couples with sexual problems. The issue of clinical relevance and utility is also considered by Derogatis and Melisaratos in their presentation of the Derogatis Sexual Function Inventory (DSFI) which focuses on the individual rather than the couple as the subject of measurement. Their article describes, in some depth, the construction of a multidimensional scale of human sexual function as well as the evaluation of its psychometric properties. Miller and Lief in the following article describe the development and application of the Sex Knowledge and Attitude Test (SKAT) which is likely the most frequently used test for the study of sexual attitudes and knowledge. The authors suggest that the value of this instrument which has been extensively used in educational settings, has not been fully realized in sex therapy research. The literature on the assessment of marital quality, adjustment and satisfaction is summarized by Spanier who discusses various conceptual problems and methodological issues dealing with the measurement of marital adjustment. The author then describes his work toward the construction and clinical application of a scale that assesses dyadic adjustment.

It is hoped that this issue will bring to the readers' attention the need for, as well as the availability of, psychological measures designed to assess the various dimensions of sexual functioning and marital interaction. These instruments not only play a significant role in the development of a scientific base for our fields of interest, but also may contribute directly to our clinical work with individuals and couples in distress.

R.C.S.

Journal of Sex & Marital Therapy
Vol. 5, No. 3, Fall 1979

The Assessment of Sexual Function and Marital Interaction

Raul C. Schiavi, MD, Leonard R. Derogatis, PhD, Judy Kuriansky, MEd, Dagmar O'Connor, MA, and Lawrence Sharpe, MD

ABSTRACT: The increasing need expressed by clinicians and researchers alike for valid and reliable psychological measures of sexual behavior and adjustment contrast with the limited available information on the assessment of human sexual functioning. The aim of this article is to present relevant data on the psychometric characteristics of scales designed to measure one or more aspects of human sexual activity and marital interaction. This list is by no means exhaustive but covers most assessments of either individuals or dyads, mainly in a heterosexual context. Under the title of the scales, which have been arranged by alphabetical order according to the first author's name, the information provided may permit a preliminary judgment concerning the potential applicability of the instrument to the reader's need.

The attempt to predict and evaluate various aspects of human behavior through the use of psychological tests has a long and varied history. DuBois has pointed out, that as far back as 1115 B.C. formal proficiency examinations were utilized by the ancient Chinese. The practices of astrology and physiognomy were embraced by the ancients as well as by more modern men, and they serve as excellent examples of man's desire to be able to predict lawfully the behavior of his fellow men.

The modern era of psychological assessment covers a much briefer period, with modern psychological evaluation resting much of its foundation on the work of three men: Alfred Binet (1905), who developed the

Dr. Schiavi is Professor of Psychiatry and Director of the Human Sexuality Program, Mount Sinai School of Medicine of the City University of New York. Dr. Derogatis is Associate Professor of Medical Psychology and Director, Division of Medical Psychology in the Department of Psychiatry, Johns Hopkins University School of Medicine, Baltimore. Ms. Kuriansky is a Clinical Intern, Department of Psychiatry, St. Luke's Hospital. Ms. O'Connor is Director, Sex Therapy Program, Department of Psychiatry, Roosevelt Hospital, New York City. Dr. Sharpe is Assistant Professor, Department of Psychiatry, Columbia Medical Center, Columbia University, New York City.

The article is based on a report prepared by the authors as members of the Research Committee of the Eastern Association for Sex Therapy (EAST, presently the Society for Sex Therapy and Research). The authors acknowledge with gratitude the support of this organization and the assistance of Ms. Natalie Weinstein in preparing the manuscript.

first practical intelligence tests; Raymond Cattell (1890), the American psychometric pioneer who created the term "mental test"; and Sir Francis Galton (1883), who was the first to develop the subject-examiner relationship so characteristic of modern psychological assessment.

To appreciate historical perspective, one should note that the first psychiatrist rating scale was developed by Kempf at Johns Hopkins in 1914, while in 1917 Robert Woodworth constructed the first self-report symptom inventory to aid in screening soldiers. At this time Rorschach was experimenting with ink blots as projective measures. The Strong Vocational Interest measure was initially published in 1927, and in 1930 Hartshorne and May first experimented with adjective checklists in the measurement of personality. The Bernreuter Personality Inventory, the first popular multidimensional personality scale, was published in 1932, and Morgan and Murray introduced the Thematic Apperception Test (TAT) in 1935. Wechsler introduced the first of his series of individual intelligence tests—The Wechsler-Bellvue Form I—in 1939. In 1943 Hathaway and McKinley published perhaps the most famous psychological test—the MMPI. Soon after, in 1944, Weider and his colleagues produced the Cornell Medical Index.

This far from exhaustive list of prominent psychological tests, is reviewed to provide a perspective for the relatively late introduction of tests measuring sexual behavior. Until the beginning of the 1960s such measures simply did not exist for all practical purposes. There was an early interest in the measurement of masculinity-femininity, which has continued and can be traced back to Terman's work in 1922. There have also been various measures of marital "adjustment," "compatibility," and the like developed through the years. The explicit domains of sexual functioning, behavior, or adjustment, however, still carried sufficient levels of societal taboo to prevent serious psychometric attempts well into the 1950s. This influence, plus the inherent complexity of human sexual behavior, have acted to delay the appearance of formal psychosexual measurement until very recently.

The principal purpose of the present report flows directly from the realization outlined above: that late application of psychometric technology in the area of human sexual behavior has resulted in a lack of general knowledge about psychological measurement in this area. Since the majority of tests designed to measure sexual behavior have been introduced during the past 10 years, the standard compendia of psychological measures often make only passing reference to them. Frequently, they are omitted entirely, since being relatively new tests their formal validation programs are often not complete.

This state of affairs exists at a time when the demand for information on valid and reliable measures which have relevance for predicting aspects of human sexual behavior is increasing at an enormous rate. The demand comes both from professionals involved in the clinical enterprise, who wish some objective manner of evaluating the impact of their treatment efforts, and from individuals engaged in research, who require valid outcome measures to evaluate the efficacies of novel and innovative treatment applications.

Our attempt here has been to compile relevant information on the psychometric characteristics of scales ostensibly designed to measure one or more aspects of human sexual activity and marital interaction. The list is by no means exhaustive, but it does cover most assessments of either individuals or dyads, mainly in a heterosexual context. Measures explicitly addressed toward homosexual or transsexual orientations have not been reviewed here.

A note should be appended concerning the posture of the authors on evaluation: we have not attempted to make any evaluative estimates concerning the "quality" or validity of the scales reviewed herein, except that a certain minimum of scientific and technical expertise was required before the instrument was considered for inclusion. In no way, however, does the inclusion of an instrument, in and of itself, signify endorsement of the instrument or agreement with its validation statements. Similarly, the omission of a specific instrument should not suggest its inadequacy. Most instruments that were included are addressed to the appropriate areas of sexual functioning, have been utilized with appropriate samples of individuals, demonstrate a reasonable level of psychometric sophistication, and show promise as sensitive, predictive reflections of human sexual behavior. Beyond this, the authors have made no evaluative judgments and maintain the position that each user should ultimately judge for oneself the merits or liabilities of any instrument described in this article.

STYLE OF THE REVIEW

A basic compilation of information has been presented under the name of each instrument and its principal author(s). An address of where the instrument may be obtained and the most relevant and descriptive literature citation has also been provided whenever possible. A synopsis of the primary objective of each instrument is given as well as the referent population and principal rater of the scale. The item format of each scale is also given; and, when available, a summary of reliability and validity information is provided.

The purpose of this particular format is to describe adequately each instrument to the reader so that one may make a preliminary judgment as to the potential applicability of each scale for one's needs. We have eschewed an evaluative format for the reason that a great deal more information would be required on each instrument and its characteristics, and in many ways it would be premature in a field where even the more established instruments have hardly had time to establish a track record.

RELIABILITY AND VALIDITY:
THEIR IMPORTANCE IN MEASUREMENT

When we speak of psychological tests, we almost always find ourselves speaking about the reliability and validity of our instruments. It is worthwhile to review these concepts briefly. Although technically the operations and concepts surrounding these two parameters of the quality of measurement can be quite complex, the basic notions of reliability and validity are really rather uncomplicated.

Reliability refers to the *consistency* with which measurement is accomplished. When it is the consistency between assessments made at two points in time, it is termed *test-retest* reliability, and is considered a measure of stability. When the consistency refers to the equality of judgments made by two raters using the same instrument, it is referred to as *interrater* reliability and is considered a measure of agreement. When consistency refers to homogeneity of items selected to measure some construct, we speak of *internal consistency* reliability. For varying types of scales these various definitions of reliability have differential importance.

The issue of validity essentially refers to the degree to which the instrument in question *actually* measures the construct(s) it purports to measure. We have known for some time that to ask, "Is the test valid?" is a meaningless interrogative, since we must ask "Valid for what purpose?" before the question can actually be answered. What is not as apparent is that there are various forms of validation, which are to a degree hierarchical, and that collectively "validation" refers to a program of studies which requires years to complete.

A basic form of validation, first described by Campbell and Fiske, has come to be called *convergent* and *discriminant* validity. Although these are two terms, they are really complementary aspects of the same concept. A demonstration of convergent validity would have the scale in question revealing high correlations with a standard accepted measure of the trait involved. Discriminant validity would reveal that the scale in question had higher correlations with the standard than with measures of other nonequivalent constructs.

Discriminant and convergent validity both fall under an older heading termed *concurrent* validity. This refers to the degree to which a scale correlates with another like-scale or other external criterion measure administered at the same time. If the criterion or standard measure is administered at a later point in time, it has been the practice in the past to refer to the level of the correlation as the degree of *predictive* validity.

The most important, and by far the most difficult form of validity to demonstrate, has come to be known as *construct* validity. This form of validation refers to a demonstration that the hypothetical construct in question is actually what is being reflected by the instrument and is at the core of what we really mean by validity. Demonstrations of all the forms of validation mentioned above all contribute to the construct validity of an instrument, and Messick has recently argued powerfully for equating the "meaning" of a measure with its construct validity. Validation is usually viewed as the more primary psychometric characteristic since it determines whether the essence of the measurement had been achieved. Reliability remains essential, however, since it places an upper ceiling on potential levels of validity.

BEYOND RELIABILITY AND VALIDITY

In addition to straightforward reliability and validity characteristics, modern psychological assessment procedures should also possess other qualities that are particularly important in modern approaches to evaluation. The first on the list, particularly in the contemporary medical or psychological setting is *brevity*. Multiple examinations, physical laboratory evaluations, lengthy treatments, and the general time limitations that are frequently seen in modern treatment settings militate against lengthy traditional methods of assessment. The psychological evaluation must be accomplished within as brief a time period as possible, and we must work to maximize the validity of brief assessment procedures rather than focus our efforts on the lengthy procedures of the past.

Second, our psychological assessment techniques must have high levels of *cost efficiency* and *cost benefit*. The former addresses the issue of whether the "cost" of the assessment procedure in terms of the time, energy, resources, and finances of the professional staff are sufficiently counterbalanced by the quality of the information derived from the evaluation to make it worthwhile. The latter characteristic addresses the question of whether the benefit accrued the patient through the application of these procedures is sufficient to justify his time, energy, and any inconvenience he may suffer as a result of the evaluation.

A third important characteristic our assessment procedures should possess is *incremental validity*. Stated most simply, incremental validity focuses on the unique contribution—actually the incremental increase in predictive power—associated with the use of a particular assessment procedure, when compared with the typical assessment techniques utilized in the clinical decision situation. If a particular assessment procedure is being considered for use in a decision situation, it should demonstrate some incremental increase in predictive validity over what is presently in use in order to qualify for inclusion. It is difficult to specify the size of a minimally acceptable increment since different clinical decisions possess inherently distinct predictive margins; nonetheless, it is particularly important in human sexual behavior that any procedure included in the assessment system be capable of a unique, valid measurement contribution.

A fourth characteristic, one that should be inherent in the design of modern assessment technique, is that of the *specific decision statement.* By this we refer to the idea that the scores, profiles, indices, or whatever the nature of the assessment summary is, be addressed to answering specific clinical decision questions rather than broad general statements concerning the patient's personality, ego functions, or psychological integration. Does the patient manifest a clinical sexual dysfunction? Is there substantial evidence for an organic etiology in this case? Are there substantial levels of marital conflict present? Is the patient's sexual experience level significantly below the norm for his age? These are the kinds of questions that form the bases of practical clinical decisions and, therefore, we believe, possess the highest predictive value for address by our assessment system in human sexual behavior. The specific decision statement represents a precise answer to a specific question concerning the patient's status. Its precision prevents waffling about our answer to the question, and its quantitative nature allows us to utilize mathematical techniques to enhance our predictive accuracy.

A final quality that we believe should be inherent in modern assessment techniques is *actuarial interpretation.* By this we mean that the assessment should be designed so that clinical interpretations are made in terms of a graduated series of norms and cutoff scores which adequately represent the populations of interest. There should also be the potential and the explicit methodology available for the development of local norms and decision-assignment values, and these should be supplied by the instrument designer.

Also, the scoring and interpretation of the measure, to the extent possible, should be in the hands of the local staff. Outside "experts" should only be utilized in an occasional consultative capacity. Systems designed to be implemented and used by local treatment staff, with occasional input from expert consultants, can go a long way toward rendering routine psychological assessment to be an effective and productive enterprise which provides important information in an efficient and uncomplicated manner.

NEGATIVE ATTITUDES TOWARD MASTURBATION SCALE
P. R. Abramson and D. L. Mosher

First Author's Address
Department of Psychology
UCLA
405 Hilgard Avenue
Los Angeles, CA 90024

Available From
Abramson PR, Mosher DL: Development of a measure of negative attitudes toward masturbation. *J Consult Clin Psychol 43*:485, 1975.

General Description
The objective of the instrument is the assessment of attitudes toward masturbation.

Subjects
Normal adults, patients with sexual dysfunctions, and psychiatric populations.

Mode of Rating
Self-report.

Items
30 items that are rated on a 5-point scale (from 1, strongly agree, to 5, strongly disagree). Examples: "When I masturbate, I am disgusted with myself"; "Masturbation is a normal, sexual outlet." A factor analysis yielded three factors: (1) positive attitude toward masturbation, (2) false beliefs about the harmful nature of masturbation, and (3) personally experienced negative affects associated with masturbation.

Reliability
Data on split-half reliability is provided in the above reference.

Validity
The authors provide validational evidence based on correlations between this measure and the average of masturbation per month for both males and females. Additional information is provided on the correlation between negative attitudes toward masturbation and sex experience and a measure of sex guilt. (See *Available From* above.)

Reference
Mosher DL, Abramson PR: Subjective sexual arousal to films of masturbation. *J Consult Clin Psychol 45*:796, 1977.

SEXUAL PLEASURE INVENTORY
J. S. Annon

Address
1481 South King Street
Honolulu, Hawaii 96814

Available From
Enabling Systems, Inc
444 Hobron Lane
Honolulu, Hawaii 96815

General Description
A checklist of people, objects, and behavior that is likely to lead to pleasure. The inventory was developed to assess the relative degree of arousal or other pleasant feelings a patient may associate with sexually related activities and experiences. A wide range of activities is covered for both sexes from the normally expected to the more rare. It can serve as a prime assessment measure for identifying and ordering specific sexual areas for therapeutic intervention.

Mode of Rating
Self-administered.

Items
Separate male and female forms with each form consisting of 130 items. Five possible responses for each item, from "not at all" to "very much" are available for each item.

Reliability
No information available.

Validity
Face validity.

Reference
Annon JS: *The Behavioral Treatment of Sexual Problems.* Vol 2, *Intensive Therapy.* Honolulu, Enabling Systems, Inc., 1976.

SEXUAL FEAR INVENTORY
J. S. Annon

Address
1481 South King Street
Honolulu, Hawaii 96814

Available From
Enabling Systems, Inc.
444 Hobron Lane
Honolulu, Hawaii 96815

General Description
(See *Sexual Pleasure Inventory.*) A self-administered checklist of people, objects, and behavior that is likely to lead to fear. There are separate male and female forms. The items

are identical to those in the Sexual Pleasure Inventory, and the same five responses are possible for each of the same 130 items. The statements concerning Sexual Pleasure Inventory apply equally to this scale.

BARRETT-LENNARD RELATIONSHIP INVENTORY
G. T. Barrett-Lennard

Address
Faculty of Arts
Department of Human Relations and Counseling Studies
University of Waterloo
Waterloo, Canada N2L 3G1

Available From
Author.

General Description
The Relationship Inventory (R-I) is a research instrument to measure four dimensions of interpersonal relationship: empathic understanding, level of regard, unconditionality, and congruence. These can be measured from the perceptions of the participants in the relationship or from the perceptions of an observer.

Subjects
Suggested for anyone with a ninth-grade education or more and can be applied in almost any situation where there is significant involvement and interaction between persons. In addition, there is a pupil form for children at sixth-grade level or above.

Mode of Rating
Ratings of A's response to B may be made by B (OS forms), by A (MO forms), or by an observer (adaptation of OS form). Four principal forms are available: (1) for reporting the other's response to self, male or female; (2) for respondent to report self-perceived response to another person, male or female; (3) experimental forms for the study of individual-group relationships; and (4) a new form to yield a representative profile of the individual's phenomenal personal environment or "relational life space." A teacher-pupil form has also been developed. Besides tapping interpersonal perceptions of "How I perceive a particular other responding to me" and "How I see my own response to the other person," changes in instructions and pronouns can yield measure of "How I think the other perceives my response to him (here)"; "How I think the other sees his (her) own response to me"; "How I would like the other to respond to me"; "How I perceive two others (or groups) responding to each other"; "How I expect others to respond to me"; or many variations or combinations of the above, at more than one stage in time, or for several categories of relationship or treatment conditions, or in association with other personality or social behavioral variables.

Items
64 items to be rated from +3 (strongly true) to −3 (strongly not true). Each of the four interpersonal variables is represented by 8 positively worded and 8 negatively worded

items. Examples: "He (she) respects me as a person"; "He (she) nearly always knows exactly what I mean"; "I nearly always feel that what he (she) says expresses exactly what he (she) is feeling and thinking as he (she) says it"; and "How much he (she) likes me is not altered by anything that I tell him (her) about myself." The items do not cover sexual topics or other particular behavioral areas.

Scoring
Answers to the 64 items yield a scale score on each of the four dimensions of interpersonal relationships.

Reliability
Test-retest and split-half reliability of the component scales have been reported to average about .85. Reliability studies have been carried out and are available from the bibliography list from the author.

Validity
Validity data is presented in an extensive bibliography available from the author. The R-I has been used in more than 100 studies examining relationships between marital clients and counselors, partners, supervisors and advisees, parents and children. The theory (Rogerian) on which this instrument was designed has been supported by other rating scales and interlocking patterns of meaningful results. This instrument's scores from perceptions of marriage partners have correlated with other measures of the adequacy of the marriage relationship. Normative data has not been collated but is available from relevant individually reported studies.

Reference
Gurman AS: The patient's perception of the therapeutic relationship. In AS Gurman, AM Razin (Eds), *Effective Psychology: A Handbook of Research.* New York, Pergamon, 1977, 503–543.

SEX-ROLE INVENTORY (SRI)
S. L. Bem

Address
Department of Psychology
Stanford University
Stanford, CA 94305

Available From
Author.

General Description
The SRI is a scale focused on the measurement of gender role definition by characterizing a person on two independent dimensions of masculinity and femininity. It also includes a social desirability scale. Masculinity and femininity scores reveal the degree of endorsement of typical masculine and feminine personality characteristics as self-descriptive. An androgeny score indicates the relative amount of masculinity and femininity that the person includes in his/her self-description.

Subjects
Adults.

Mode of Rating
Self-report.

Items
60 descriptive personality characteristics rated on 7-point Likert scales.

Reliability
Both test-retest and internal consistency reliability reported in reference publications.

Validity
Validation studies reported in reference publications.

References
Bem S: The measurement of psychological androgyny. *J Consult Clin Psychol 42*:155, 1974.
Bem S: Sex-role adaptability: One consequence of psychological androgyny. *J Pers Soc Psychol 31*:634, 1975.

HETEROSEXUAL BEHAVIOR ASSESSMENTS
P. M. Bentler

Address
Department of Psychology
University of California
Los Angeles, CA 90024

Available From
Author.

General Description
The objective of the instrument is the assessment of heterosexual behaviors. The scale can be used as a hierarchy in desensitization therapy or can be applied to the assessment of behavioral change resulting from therapy. There are two versions: one for males and the other for females, in both long and short forms.

Subjects
Adults.

Mode of Rating
Self-report.

Items
A Guttman-type scale, consisting of 21 classes of heterosexual behaviors arranged in hierarchical manner. The number of items endorsed by the subject provides the total score. Several items are specific to either the male or female.

Reliability and Validity

Psychometric evaluation of the scale assessed in a college-educated population indicated satisfactory scalability and internal consistency. Short 10-item forms for males or females which correlate .98 with a total scale are available.

References

Bentler PM: Heterosexual behavior assessments I. Males. *Behav Res Ther* 6:21, 1968.
Bentler PM: Heterosexual behavior assessment II. Females. *Behav Res Ther* 6:27, 1968.

A MARITAL COMMUNICATION INVENTORY
M. J. Bienvenu, Sr.

Address

Family Life Publications, Inc.
P. O. Box 427
Saluda, NC 28773

Available From

Address above.

General Description

The Marital Communication Inventory (MCI) is a questionnaire that has been designed to provide an objective measure of success or failure in marital communication.

Subjects

Couples.

Mode of Rating

Self-report.

Items

46 items with four responses to each question: usually, sometimes, seldom, and never, which are scored from 0 to 3 with a favorable response (the one indicative of good communication) given the higher score.

Reliability

A split-half correlation coefficient revealed a corrected coefficient of .93.

Validity

A comparison of the scores obtained from a group receiving marital counseling and a matched group without apparent marital problems revealed a significant difference in marital communication in favor of the group without apparent problems.

Reference

Bienvenue MJ, Sr: Measurement of marital communication. *Fam Coordinator 19*:26, 1970.

SELF-DISCLOSURE QUESTIONNAIRE
A. M. Bodin

Address
Mental Research Institute
555 Middlefield Road
Palo Alto, CA 94301

Available From
Author

General Description
The purpose of this questionnaire is the assessment of self-disclosure to spouse and of the perceived disclosure from the spouse on various aspects of living, including (1) personality, (2) body and health, (3) childhood and family, and (4) marital relationship. This instrument is a revised version of the self-disclosure questionnaire of Sidney Jourard.

Subjects
Couples.

Mode of Rating
Self-report.

Items
52 items to be rated on an 8-point scale of how much he or she has revealed himself (herself) to the spouse about the topic of each item and how he or she thinks the spouse will respond to the same item. The extremes of the scale are (1) "I have revealed myself to this person about this topic incorrectly by intentionally misrepresenting myself in order to give a false picture of me" and (8) "I have revealed myself to this person about this topic completely and without any reservations whatsoever." Sample items: "What it takes to hurt my feelings deeply . . ."; "What I dislike most about my spouse as a lover[.] . . ." The couple is asked to complete the questionnaire separately and independently.

Validity and Reliability
No information on validity or reliability is available.

Reference
Comrey AL, Backer TE, Glaser, EM (Eds): *A Source Book for Mental Health Measures.* Los Angeles, Human Interaction Research Institute, 1973, p. 187.

THE DEROGATIS SEXUAL FUNCTION INVENTORY (DSFI)
Leonard R. Derogatis

Address
Henry Phipps Clinic
Johns Hopkins Hospital
Baltimore, MD 21205

Available From
Author.

General Description

The DSFI is an omnibus-type scale designed to reflect accurately levels of current sexual functioning. The unit of measurement for the DSFI is the individual. The DSFI measures sexual functioning via eight major domains of sexual functioning, and a corresponding subtest for each: I. Information, II. Experience, III. Drive, IV. Attitudes, V. Symptoms, VI. Affect, VII. Gender Role Definition, VIII. Fantasy, IX. Body Image, and X. Satisfaction. Scores on each of the subtests are first standardized and then summed to provide a single summary score (the DSFI Score) which communicates the individual's overall level of sexual functioning.

Subjects

Adults.

Mode of Rating

Self-report.

Items

245 separate items which require approximately 30 to 40 minutes for the patient to complete. In addition, there is a single 9-point Global Sexual Satisfaction Index which provides a measure of the patient's self-rating of his/her present level of sexual functioning.

Two of the subtests of the DSFI are themselves distinct psychological measuring instruments that may be scored and displayed in a multidimensional fashion. Symptoms are reflected by the Brief Symptom Inventory (BSI) which may be scored in terms of nine primary symptom dimensions plus three global indices: somatization, obsessive-compulsive, interpersonal sensitivity, depression, anxiety, hostility, phobic anxiety, paranoid ideation, and psychoticism plus the three global measures. Similarly, affect is reflected by the Affect Balance Scale (ABS) which reflects the patient's current mood state in terms of eight affect dimensions—four positive and four negative—plus three global or summary measures: joy, contentment, vigor, affection, anxiety, depression, guilt and hostility plus the Affect Balance Index and positive and negative affect totals.

Reliability and Validity

At present provisional norms are available for the DSFI. These consist of data on 200 normal individuals, plus analogous data on approximately 200 sexually dysfunctional individuals. The file is being continually updated, and it is anticipated that normative groups double this size will soon be available. In addition, an extensive presentation of psychometric and validation information in a formal manual is presently being completed.

References

Derogatis LR: Psychological assessment of the sexual disabilities. In JK Meyer (Ed), *The Clinical Management of Sexual Disorders.* Baltimore, Williams & Wilkins, 1976.

Derogatis LR, Meyer JK, Dupkin C: Discrimination of psychogenic versus organic impotence with the DSFI. *J Sex Marital Ther 2*:229, 1976.

Derogatis LR, Meyer JK, Gallant BW: Distinctions between male and female invested partners in sexual disorders. *Am J Psychiatry 134*:385, 1977.

Derogatis LR, Meyer JK, Vazquez N: A psychological profile of the transsexual: 1. The male. *J Nerv Ment Dis 166*:234, 1978.

THE SEXUAL ORIENTATION METHOD
M. P. Feldman, M. J. MacCulloch, V. Mellor, and J. M. Pinschof

First Author's Address
Department of Psychology
University of Birmingham
Elms Road, P.O. Box 363
Birmingham, B15 2TT, England

Available From
Feldman MP, MacCulloch MJ, et al: The application of anticipatory avoidance learning to the treatment of homosexuality. III. The sexual orientation method. *Behav Res Ther* 4:289, 1966.

General Description
This is a questionnaire aimed at assessing the relative degree of homo- and heteroerotic orientation of men who show homosexual behavior. It is derived from the Semantic Differential Technique of Osgood. The questionnaire may be used to evaluate the response of homosexual patients to treatment, but it is not intended to detect homosexuality in subjects who are not known to have homosexual characteristics.

Subjects
Adult men.

Mode of Rating
Self-report.

Items
Questions presented at random in pairs with a total of 120 pairs. Pairs 1–60 concern attitudes to males and 61–120 concern attitudes to women. The subjects are asked to respond with one of six adjectives (interesting, attractive, handsome, hot, pleasurable, and exciting) to two concepts: "Men are sexually to me..." and "Women are sexually...." Five scale positions are used for each adjective, e.g., (1) very attractive, (2) quite attractive, (3) neither attractive nor unattractive, (4) quite unattractive, and (5) very unattractive.

Reliability
Data is presented in the article cited under Available From showing that this assessment method has adequate internal consistency and unidimensionality. Test-retest reliability in samples of control subjects ranged between 0.80 and 0.94.

Validity
Pretreatment mean scores of homosexual patients were found to be significantly different from control groups. The scores following aversion therapy for homosexuality were significantly related to independent assessment of clinical improvement.

Reference
Sambrooks, JE, MacCulloch MJ: A modification of the sexual orientation method and automated technique for presentation and scoring. *Br J Soc Clin Psychol 12*:163, 1973. (A revision of the Sexual Orientation Method.)

SEXUAL COMPATIBILITY TEST
A. L. Foster

Address
The Phoenix Institute of California
248 Blossom Hill Road
Los Gatos, CA 95030

Available From
Address above.

General Description
A test for the assessment of sexual attitudes, activity, responsiveness, and satisfaction in couples.

Subjects
For use in couples presenting with sexual problems. Of some use in couples presenting with other psychodynamic difficulties.

Mode of Rating
Self-administered test. It can be presented individually or to groups. No special training is required for administration of the test.

Items
64 items. Each item questions specific sexual activity involving the couple and demands answers along six separate dimensions. A further 37 items require single responses to each specific question. Scoring can be computerized. Programs are available on many dimensions including satisfaction-dissatisfaction as a couple, sexual activity, desired sexual activity, pleasure, etc. Seven major scales assess overall sexual functioning: activity level, desired activity level, pleasure, perception of mate's pleasure, desired pleasure, desire for mate's pleasure, and sexual problem-solving skills. Six scales assess the type and degree of sexual dysfunctioning. Twelve subscales measure specific sexual activities and feelings and attitudes about those activities: nudity, embracing, loving verbalizations, kissing, oral-genital, manual-genital, intercourse activities, caressing, and sexual variety. All scales can be profiled for clear visualization. A scale with cutoff scores predicting the likelihood of success in treating a couple's sexual problems is also available.

Reliability and Validity
Studies are reported to have been done but are unpublished.

References
Foster AL: Manual of Sexual Compatibility Test. Los Gatos, CA, 1974. The Phoenix Institute of California.
Foster AL: The Sexual Compatibility Test. *J. Consult Clin Psychol*, 45:332, 1977.
Foster AL, Gianatasio J, Kelly CA: *Matching validity study of the Sexual Compatibility Test.* Unpublished manuscript, 1975.
Southern ML: Concurrent validity of Sexual Compatibility Test. Unpublished manuscript, 1975.

SEXUALITY EXPERIENCE SCALES (SES)
J. Frenken

Address

Dutch Institute for Social Sexological Research
Zeist, Whilhelminalaan 5
The Netherlands

Available From

Author.

General Description

An inventory of various aspects of sexual behavior and experience. It was constructed as a measurement instrument for (group) research, not for individual diagnostic use. It can be used in different kinds of research, e.g., survey studies on sexual behavior and attitudes, marriage research, and as an outcome instrument in research in sexual dysfunction therapy.

Development

Theoretical consideration led to the formulation of a hypothetical basic dimension of sexual experience: acceptance versus rejection of sexuality. This was operationalized in 182 verbal self-report questions and statements about own experience and administered to a random stratified pilot group of married middle-class Dutch men and women up to 50 years of age. Item selection identified 76 items, found by factor analysis to belong to three factors: traditional restrictive sex morals (acceptance v. rejection), psychosexual stimulation (seeking, allowing/avoidance, rejection), and sexual motivation (appetitive v. aversive). A measure was further constructed for the degree of attraction to marriage (as marriage was found to be a relevant variable).

Mode of Rating

Self-report.

Items

83 multiformated questions. Example: "Some women have very little need of intercourse. Others have a strong need. How often would you prefer to have intercourse? (1), Less than once a month; (2), Once a month; (3) 2–3 times a month; (4) Once a week; (5), 2–3 times a week; and (6) 4 or more times a week."

Reliability

Reliabilities for the four scales varied from .86 to .92 with a mean of .89.

Validity

Internal consistency of the four scales was found to be adequate. Construct validity was established for the following hypotheses: (1) The more a person accepts a restrictive moral attitude to sex, the stronger his aversion to and inhibition in sexual behavior. (2) The more a person accepts a restrictive sex moral, the stronger his rejection of psychosexual stimulation induced by internal and external criteria and the stronger his tendency to increased inhibition of sexual behavioral responses to these stimuli. (3) The stronger a person's rejection of psychosexual stimulation, the stronger his aversion of sexual responses. (4) The stronger a person's aversion of sexual behavior with a partner, the lower his attraction to marriage. (5) The lower a person's attraction-to-marriage, the stronger his seeking for psychosexual stimulation induced by internal and external stimuli as a means of vicarious gratification.

The relationship between the sex constructs and other personality variables measured by 8 personality inventories is being explored (e.g. FIRO scales, Rokeach Dogmatism Scale).

Usefulness
SES can be used in intake interview with patients when exact value of the score is not stressed. The scales give some insight on specific problems in sex matters by looking at answers on individual items. Specific item ratings can be discussed with the patient (e.g., "What did you mean with your answer 'very unpleasant' on this item?") to help set up a therapy strategy for that patient. Scores also give an indication (albeit somewhat arbitrary) of where patient stands in a normative continuum (i.e., in which quarter of the frequency distribution).

Reference
Frenken J: *Sexuality Experience Scales.* Amsterdam, Swets and Zeitlinger, in press.

SEX ATTITUDE QUESTIONNAIRE
B. Fretz

Address
Department of Psychology
University of Maryland
College Park, MD 20742

Available From
Author.

General Description
A brief self-report measure of attitudes toward behaviors and situations broadly con-strued as sexual in our society. It can be used to measure the degree of positive or negative regard for sexual behaviors among specific populations and to assess the effects of pertinent communications such as sex education on attitude change. There are both long and short forms of concepts, each evaluated along bipolar dimensions (semantic differential).

Subjects
Males or females with or without sexual or other problems.

Mode of Rating
Self-report.

Items
The initial long-form semantic differential consisted of 30 concepts each with 17 bipolar dimensions (510 responses). Concepts were chosen to represent the full spectrum of

behaviors identified as sexual in our society. Dimensions were chosen from existing literature employing the semantic differential. Factor analyses of this form administered to 128 college students and 154 teachers revealed four factors: the evaluative factor; a combination of the potency and activity factors (as previously identified by Osgood and now referred to as a dynamism factor); the understanding factor; and a fourth factor which was not readily interpretable. Further factor analyses identified 10 relatively independent *concepts* and 7 *factors*.

The final short form includes: 12 concepts each evaluated on seven bipolar dimensions. Evaluative dimensions include good-bad, valuable-worthless, kind-cruel. Understanding dimensions include understandable-mysterious and familiar-strange. Dynamic dimensions include active-passive and fast-slow. The factor structure of the revised measure, administered to a new group of 97 college students, essentially replicated the structure of the longer measure. Concepts in the shortened form, however, were not as empirically independent as in the long form.

Scoring
Items can be scored on scale from 1 to 7; or changes noted in subject's response at two points in time.

Reliability
The retest reliability of the short form on bipolar dimensions ranged from .78 (good-bad) to .52 (active-passive). Test-retest reliability by concept ranged from .35 for homosexual to .67 for the oral and/or anal intercourse concept. Reliabilities in the short form were generally lower than in the long form.

Validity
Evidence of external validity has been provided in studies using one instrument to evaluate the effects of sex education programs revealing significant pre-post treatment changes. Attitudes toward certain concepts changed more frequently than others. Ratings of dynamic dimensions show the least change; ratings of evaluative dimensions, the most change. Intergroup comparisons (i.e., teachers, students, parents, nurses) failed to support existing stereotypes. (For example, neither the beginning nursing students nor the parent sample showed the negative rating patterns that had been expected on some of the more "taboo" concepts, and university students did not show positive halo ratings that the stereotype of the sexually active promiscuous student culture would imply.) The *least* positive ratings across all concepts and dimensions were generally given by the teacher sample; the most positive ratings occurred with about equal frequency among student and parent samples. The measure is currently being used in a longitudinal study of university student attitudes as there is a trend, suggested in the ratings from freshmen and seniors, toward more positive ratings among upper classmen.

References
Bekander I: Semantic description of complex and meaningful stimulus material. *Percep Mot Skills* 22:201, 1966.
Fretz BR: An attitude measure of sexual behaviors. Paper presented at the American Psychological Association, 1974.
Nunnally JC: *Popular Conceptions of Mental Health.* New York: Holt, 1961.
Osgood C, Suci G, Tannenbaum P: *The Measurement of Meaning.* Urbana, University of Illinois Press, 1957.

BIOGRAPHICAL MARITAL QUESTIONNAIRE
B. L. Greene

Address
University of Illinois School of Medicine
Chicago, IL

Available From
Greene BL: *A Clinical Approach to Marital Problems.* Springfield, Ill., Thomas, 1970.

General Description
This questionnaire originally developed by Maholick and Shapiro was modified by
Greene for the systematic gathering of information on couples with marital disharmony.
Its central aim is to obtain background data about the couple, as well as information on
the affectional aspects of the marriage, feelings about kinship networks, divisions of
responsibility in the home, and what each spouse views as a major source of difficulty.
Greene utilized this questionnaire to gather data on 750 couples with marital problems
from his private practice as well as from a marital clinic. The results obtained by this
questionnaire have been organized and presented in the above-mentioned book.

Subjects
Couples.

Mode of Rating
Self-report.

Items
22 open-ended questions requiring narrative responses. Each partner is instructed to
complete it independently providing as much information as he/she considers necessary
to answer each item. Sample question: "What are your specific complaints about your
marriage? (First circle and then describe.) (a) Lack of communication; (b) Constant argu-
ments; (c) Unfulfilled emotional needs; (d) Sexual dissatisfaction; (e) Financial dis-
agreements; (f) In-law trouble; (g) Infidelity; (h) Conflicts about children; (i) Domineer-
ing spouse; (j) Suspicious spouse, and (k) Others."

Reliability and Validity
No data are currently available.

Reference
Greene BL: *A clinical Approach to Marital Problems.* Springfield, Ill., Thomas, 1970.

A QUESTIONNAIRE MEASURE OF SEXUAL INTEREST
J. J. M. Harbison, P. J. Graham, J. T. Quinn,
H. McAllister, and R. Woodward

First Author's Address
Departments of Mental Health, Psychology, and Social Studies
The Queen's University of Belfast
Belfast, Ireland

Available From
First author.

General Description
The aim of this questionnaire is to measure the degree of interest the male or female indicates in particular sexual situations which might be of either homosexual or heterosexual nature. This instrument is derived from the Sexual Orientation Method of Feldman et al. The test is relatively long to complete and to score unless computer facilities are available. It may be applicable to assess differences in sexual interest between clinical and normal groups or to monitor the response of patients to treatment.

Subjects
Adults.

Mode of Rating
Self-report.

Items
140 items set out in random order, and the subject is told to mark the adjectival statement that best describes his/her response to the sexual situation in question. Five different aspects of sexual behavior are measured (kissing, being kissed, touching sexually, being touched sexually, and sexual intercourse) along four bipolar adjectival scales (seductive-repulsive, sexy-sexless, exciting-dull, and erotic-frigid). Five scale positions are used for each adjective, e.g., (a) very erotic, (b) quite erotic, (c) neither erotic nor frigid, (d) quite frigid and (e) very frigid.

Reliability and Validity
Preliminary data on internal consistency, test-retest reliability, and validity are reported in the reference below.

Reference
Harbison JJM et al: A Questionnaire Measure of Sexual Interest. *Arch Sex Behav 3*:357, 1974.

BODY CONTACT QUESTIONNAIRE
M. H. Hollender

Address
Department of Psychiatry
Vanderbilt Medical Center
Nashville, TENN 37232

Available From
Author.

General Description
This instrument has been developed to assess the desire for body contact.

Subjects
Adults.

Mode of Rating
Self-report.

Items
12 items scored on a 5-point Likert Scale. Sample question: "If you have trouble falling asleep, it is helpful to have someone hold you." The scoring is done on the basis of "never" (1) and "always" (5). The minimum score is, therefore, 12, and the maximum score is 60.

Reliability
When questions about the wish to be held were tested for internal consistency, the reliability coefficient was .82. A test-retest reliability coefficient of .94 indicated that the scores on two occasions were approximately the same.

Validity
No information is available.

References
Hollender MH, Luborsky L, Scavamella TJ: Body contact and sexual excitement. *Arch Gen Psychiatry 20*:188, 1969.
Hollender MH, Mercer AJ: Wish to be held and wish to hold in men and women. *Arch Gen Psychiatry 33*:49, 1976.

SEXUAL AROUSABILITY INVENTORY (FEMALE FORM)
E. F. Hoon, P. W. Hoon, and J. P. Wincze

First Author's Address
College of Medicine, Department of Psychiatry
The University of Tennessee
865 Poplar
Memphis, TENN 38104

Available From
First author.

General Description
This is a pencil-and-paper inventory of sexual arousability for women. The inventory consists of descriptions of sexual activities and situations. The respondent rates each on a 7-point Likert scale on the basis of how sexually arousing the described activity is to her.

Subjects
Females.

Mode of Rating
Self-report.

Items
28 descriptions. Sample items: "When you hear sounds of pleasure during sex...";
"When a loved one undresses you...." The extremes of the scale are −1 ("adversely affects arousal; unthinkable, repulsive, distracting") and 5 ("always causes sexual arousal; extremely arousing"). A total score is obtained by (1) adding positive scores, (2) adding

negative scores, and (3) subtracting the sum of any negative scores from the sum of positive scores. A factor analysis resulted in five basic dimensions of erotic arousability. The factor loadings may be obtained by writing to the first author.

Reliability and Validity

The authors report data showing that the instrument has adequate stability and internal consistency. Concurrent validity was evaluated in relation to reported awareness of physiological changes of sexual arousal, sexual satisfaction, and frequency of intercourse. The instrument was cross-validated with the Bentler Heterosexual Experience Scale. The norms provided are derived from the validation and cross-validation samples comprised of women of middle and upper middle socioeconomic classes. Norms are available from the first author. They include an additional sample of 85 women, 25 years or older. The norms of the new total sample ($N = 370$) including additional data from older women remain essentially the same as the originally published norms. The instrument discriminated between a sample of normal females and a group of women seeking therapy for sexual dysfunctions.

Reference

Hoon EF, Hoon PW, Wincze JP: An inventory for the measurement of female sexual arousability: The SAI. *Arch Sex Behav* 5:291, 1976.

INDEX OF MARITAL SATISFACTION (IMS)
W. W. Hudson

Address

School of Social Work
University of Hawaii
Honolulu, Hawaii 96822

Available From

Author.

General Description

A short scale measuring the degree or magnitude of discord or dissatisfaction (but not source or cause) that partners experience with the interpersonal component of their relationship. The scale is designed as part of a set of seven short-form measurement scales collectively referred to as the Clinical Measurement Package, designed to monitor, guide, and evaluate clinical treatment.

Subjects

Adults.

Mode of Rating

Self-rating.

Items

25 items, both positively and negatively worded (to partially control for response bias). Examples: "I feel that my partner really cares for me"; "I feel that we should do more things together."

Scoring

Subject rates items along a 5-point continuum from 1 (rarely or none of the time) to 5 (most or all of the time). Positively stated items are then reversed scored so all low scores indicate relative absence of problem. A clinical cutting score of 30 has been established as a diagnostic benchmark and a criterion for treatment effectiveness. With multiple administration, data records can be used to form time-lines tracing the impact of treatment on the severity of the problem and supplemented with notations about critical incidents.

Reliability

In the range of .90.

Validity

Established and reported in papers available from the author.

Reference

Hudson WW: A measurement package for clinical workers. Unpublished manuscript.

INDEX OF SEXUAL SATISFACTION (ISS)
W. W. Hudson

Address

School of Social Work
University of Hawaii
Honolulu, Hawaii 96822

Available From

Author.

General Description

A short scale measuring the degree or magnitude of discord or dissatisfaction (but not source or cause) that partners experience with the sexual component of their relationship. It is designed as part of a set of seven short-form measurement scales collectively referred to as the Clinical Measurement Package, designed to monitor, guide, and evaluate clinical treatment.

Subjects

Adults.

Mode of Rating

Self-rating.

Items

25 items, both positively and negatively worded. Examples: "My sex life is very exciting"; "My partner does not want sex when I do."

Reference

Hudson WW, Glisson D: *A Short-form Scale to Measure Sexual Dissatisfaction.* Honolulu, University of Hawaii School of Social Work, 1976.

MARITAL COMMUNICATION SCALE (MCS)
M. Kahn

Address
University of Miami, Florida
P.O. Box 8186
Coral Gables, FLA 33124

Available From
Author.

General Description
This scale is a situational measure of nonverbal communication accuracy which permits free response by the expresser but is still scored objectively. The MCS requires mates to communicate a standard set of messages to each other in a dyadic, face-to-face setting. Each item includes the following parts: a hypothetical situation which calls for a communication from one spouse to the other; three possible attitudes or intentions regarding this situation and a specific verbal message. For each item the message is developed so that it can conceivably imply all three of the attitudes or intentions accompanying the given situation. The object is for the expresser to communicate to his partner through the verbal message the alternative intention that has been designated by the experimenter. Since the content is fixed and can imply all three of the intentions, the expresser's only means of providing the receiver with the necessary discrimination is through the use of nonverbal cues. After each communication is completed, the receiver is given a copy of the three alternative intentions for that item and must select the one that he believes his partner had attempted to convey.

Subjects
Couples.

Items
16 items. For 8 items the husband is the expresser and the wife the receiver, while the roles are reversed for the remaining items. The score is the total number of items accurately communicated with a possible range of 0 to 16. The combined scores are used since each item requires the contributions of both spouses.

Reliability
Data in split-half reliability and test-retest reliability can be obtained from the author.

Validity
In one study MCS scores have discriminated between satisfied and dissatisfied couples.

Reference
Kahn M: Non-verbal communication and marital satisfaction. *Fam Process 9*:449, 1970.

BODY ATTITUDE SCALE
R. Kurtz and M. Hirt

First Author's Address
Department of Psychology
Washington University
St. Louis, MO 63130

Available From
First author.

General Description
A self-report scale that measures global attitudes toward the outward form of a person's body on three primary attitude dimensions. Thirty different body concepts (or parts) are rated on a modification of the Osgood semantic differential.

Subjects
Adults of various ages and backgrounds with or without physical or psychological disorders.

Items
Samples of items: "size of my arms," "color of my hair," "size of my bust." There are no specific sexual concepts rated.

Mode of Ratings
Ratings are made on a 7-point bipolar adjective scale sampling, three dimensions of the Osgood's semantic differential: evaluative (good-bad); potency (strong-weak); and activity (active-passive).

Scoring
A 7-point scale is used with 1 being the most negative, 4 neutral, and 7 the most positive. The three adjectival scales for each dimension are then summed to obtain an "item" score for each concept on each dimension. These item scores can then be summed across the 30 body concepts to obtain a composite global body attitude score. This can be done for each dimension separately, yielding an evaluative body attitude score, a potency body attitude score, and an activity body attitude score.

Reliability
Available from author.

Validity
Evidence for internal consistency of the body attitude measures has been reported. The generalizability coefficients for both males and females ranged from .93 to .98 on all three dimensions, indicating that attitudes toward the postulated universe of global body attitudes could be inferred adequately from their specific attitudes toward individual body aspects. It has also been shown that chronically ill subjects evaluate their bodily appearance more negatively than normal subjects, with regard to the evaluative and activity dimensions.

References
Hirt M, Kurtz R. A re-examination of the relationship between body boundary and site of disease. *J Abnorm Psychol 74*:67, 1969.
Hirt M, Ross WD, Kurtz R, Gleser G: Attitudes to body products among normal subjects. *J Abnorm Psychol 74*:486, 1969.
Kurtz R, The relationship of body attitude to sex, body size and body build in a college population. *Dissert Abstracts 6*:27, 1966.
Kurtz R, Hirt M: Body attitude and physical health. *J Clin Psychol 26*:149, 1970.

THE FOUR RELATIONSHIP FACTOR QUESTIONNAIRE
G. F. Lawlis

Address
Department of Psychology
North Texas State University
Denton, TX 76203

Available From
Test Systems, Inc.
P.O. Box 18432
Wichita, KA 67218

General Description
This is a self-report questionnaire to identify the perceptions of people's relationships in a wide range of interactions. It is filled out by an individual with reference to his perception of a specific relationship with another individual.

Subjects
All age ranges above third-grade reading levels. The scale has most often been used with children and their parents and teachers, between parents, and client's with their counselors. Marriage counselors have found it useful in determining mental problems, and vocational counselors have used the test to determine difficulties in client's rehabilitation training problems.

Development and Norms
Originally, the questionnaire was standardized on 200 normals. Then an additional 200 children and adults were added to the distribution. Currently, new norms are being collected for deviate groups, such as juvenile delinquents, abusive parents, and alcoholics.

Items
44 items rated as (1) always true, (2) sometimes true, (3) sometimes false, or (4) always false. Items are short statements. Examples in the sexul factor: "I like her/him to touch me"; "He/She can turn me on"; "She/He is sexy"; "I love him/her." The sex factor relates to both the sexual and affectional aspect of the relationship, i.e., how one is "turned on" emotionally as a function of being with the other person. Examples of other items: "I respect his/her standards"; "We think a lot alike"; "I like to work with him/her on projects." The four factors, or dimensions of relationships are not meant to imply pathology or level of maturity, but rather to represent the mode of interaction between two people.

Scoring
A weight from 0 to 3 is automatically recorded for each response. Scoring is fast and can be done by the testee.

Reliability
Intratest reliabilities are between .69 and .81 on 100 adult subjects for the four factors; test-retest reliabilities are between .91 and .98 on 28 adults.

Validity
Various studies of concurrent and predictive validity are described in the test manual. For example; the test factors correlated .95 with the nature of the relationship (friend, mate,

etc.). Also, case profiles predicted treatment outcome, and children's relation with parents predicted academic performance at a significant level.

References

The following dissertations are available from Texas Tech. Dissertations, Lubbock, Texas: Waters G: *Marriage Relationships;* Norman B: *Dynamic Personality and Relationships;* Tom G: *School Achievement and Parental Relationships.*

Other references in *Psychological Reports* and *Forensic Psychology* are available from author.

SEX KNOWLEDGE AND ATTITUDE TEST (SKAT)
H. I. Lief and D. M. Reed

First Author's Address
Division of Family Study
Department of Psychiatry
University of Pennsylvania School of Medicine
4025 Chestnut Street
Philadelphia, PA 19104

Available From
First author.

General Description
The SKAT is a scale oriented toward the gathering of information about sexual attitudes, sexual knowledge, and the level of experience in sexual activities. A certain amount of demographic and biographical data is also collected. It is an omnibus-type scale designed to function as both a teaching aid and a research instrument in human sexuality. The SKAT is comprised of 149 items in four distinct areas: attitudes, knowledge, demography and sexual experiences. The scale takes approximately 30 minutes to complete.

Subjects
Adults.

Mode of Rating
Self-report.

Type of Items
Multiple choice.

Reliability
Internal consistency coefficients in the 70s and 80s and test-retest coefficients in the 80s reported in a preliminary manual.

Validity
Numerous validity studies are reported in the manual.

Reference
Preliminary technical manual available from the first author.

LOCKE-WALLACE MARRIAGE INVENTORY
H. J. Locke and K. M. Wallace

Available From

Locke HJ, Wallace KM: Short marital adjustment and prediction tests: Their reliability and validity. *Marr Fam Living 21*:251, 1959. A modified form of Locke's Marital Questionnaire and scoring key is reproduced in D Kimmel, F Van der Veen, Factors of marital adjustment. *J Marr Fam 36*:57, 1974.

General Description

This inventory provides a measure of marital adjustment covering marital adjustment and satisfaction. It was originally developed by Locke who proposed a 29-item test designed to discriminate between "successful" and "unsuccessful" marriages. In 1959 Locke and Wallace published a shortened form of this test, which has been frequently used for the assessment of marital adjustment. Recently, Kimmel and Van der Veen published a revised version of the original Locke Marital Adjustment Questionnaire. It has the 23 most significant items with scores weighed to reflect current sex differences in patterns of responding.

Subjects

Couples.

Mode of Rating

Self-report.

Items

Locke and Wallace form—15 items concerning how husbands and wives perceive or assess their marriage. The items have several formats: Some of the items have multiple-choice responses such as "Have you ever wished you had not married? (a) Frequently; (b) Occasionally; (c) Rarely." Other items ask the extent of agreement or disagreement in marital issues such as "ways of dealing with in-laws"; responses to these items are checked on a 6-point scale from "always agree" to "always disagree." One item consists of 22 areas of potentially serious difficulties of which the respondent checks as many as is applicable. The last item provides a 7-point scale from "very unhappy" to "perfectly happy" with the following instruction: "On the scale line below check the mark which best describes the degree of happiness, everything considered, of your marriage." Responses are scored according to a system of weighted scores described by Locke.

Reliability

The Locke and Wallace standard form had a reliability of .90 computed by the split-half technique. Kimmel and Van der Veen conducted a factor analytic study on the husband and wife's separate scores of the 23-item version of the Locke Marital Adjustment Questionnaire. It was found that the instrument is an internally consistent measure of marital adjustment and that it consists of two separate components labeled "sexual congeniality" and "compatibility." The scores for each factor were found to be stable over a 2-year test-retest interval.

Validity

The Locke and Wallace form was reported as a valid measure since it was able to discriminate between well adjusted and maladjusted couples with a minimal overlap in the range of scores between the two groups.

References
See *Available From.*
Locke HJ: *Predicting Adjustment in Marriage: A Comparison of a Divorced and a Happily Married Group,* New York, Holt, 1951.
Locke H, Williamson RC: Marital adjustment: A factor analysis study. *Am Soc Rev 23* :562, 1958.

THE SEXUAL INTERACTION INVENTORY
J. LoPiccolo and J. C. Steger

First Author's Address
Department of Psychiatry and Behavioral Science
State University of New York at Stony Brook
Stony Brook, NY 11790

Available From
First author.

General Description
This is an inventory for the assessment of sexual adjustment and sexual satisfaction of heterosexual couples.

Subjects
Couples.

Mode of Rating
Self-report.

Items
A list of 17 items covering a wide range of heterosexual behaviors. For each behavior both husband and wife answer independently 6 questions on a 6-point rating scale. The totals from each member of the couple are used to derive an 11-scale profile. The scales assess (1) degree of satisfaction with the frequency and range of sexual behaviors for the male and female respectively, (2) self-acceptance regarding the pleasure derived from engaging in sexual activities, (3) pleasure obtained from sexual activity, (4) accuracy of knowledge of partner's preferred sexual activities, and (5) degree of acceptance of partner. The last scale is an overall summary scale. Approximately 30 to 40 minutes are required for the completion of the scale. The author has developed a computer program which scores optical scan answer sheets and lists critical items.

Reliability
Test-retest reliability values range from .67 to .90 for the 11 scales. These correlations have been significant at the .05 level or better with a sample size of 15. The authors have also provided data on internal consistency.

Validity
The convergent and discriminant validity of the instrument has been assessed. The Sexual Interaction Inventory discriminated between couples suffering from sexual dysfunctions and sexually satisfied couples. Longitudinal data is reported indicating that all 11

scales of the Sexual Interaction inventory reflect changes induced by therapy in a group of patients suffering from sexual dysfunctions.

References

LoPiccolo J, Steger JC: The Sexual Interaction Inventory: A new instrument for assessment of sexual dysfunction. *Arch Sex Behav 3*:585, 1974.
McGovern KB, Stewart RC, and LoPiccolo J: Secondary orgasmic dysfunction. I. Analysis and strategies for treatment. *Arch Sex Behav 4:*265, 1975.

SEX-ROLE SURVEY
A. P. MacDonald, Jr.

Address
Director
University of Wisconsin System-wide Center
for the Study of Minorities and the Disadvantaged
Office of the Graduate School
P.O. Box 413
University of Wisconsin-Milwaukee
Milwaukee, WI 53201

Available From
Publications Office
Center for the Study of Human Sexuality
4105 Medical Parkway, Suite 205
Austin, TX 78756

General Description
A self-report scale measuring subject's attitudes toward sex roles.

Subjects
Ranging in age from 14 to 73 years of age of various educational and social-class levels.

Mode of Rating
Self-report.

Items
53 items, though a 20-item short form available. Example: "As head of the household, the father should have final authority over children."

Scoring
Each item is scored by the subject on a 9-point scale of agreement ranging from "I agree very much" through "I disagree very much." Scores yield a total score and four factors: (1) equality in business and the professions, (2) sex-role appropriate behavior, (3) equal involvement in social and domestic work, and (4) power in the home.

Reliability
On a study of 317 males and 322 females, ranging in age from 14 to 73, alpha coefficients on the four factors and total score were obtained as follows: (1) business and the profes-

sions: .94; (2) sex-role appropriate behavior: .85; (3) social and domestic work: .85; (4) power in the home: .86; and (5) SRS total: .96.

Validity
Normative data and information on validity is supplied in the references. The instrument has been used in the school system of Rochester, New York.

References
MacDonald AP, Jr, Games RG: Some characteristics of those who hold positive and negative attitudes toward homosexuals. *J Homosex 1*:9, 1974.
MacDonald AP, Jr: Identification and measurement of multidimensional attitudes toward equality between the sexes. *J Homosex 1*:165, 1974.

ATTITUDES TOWARD HOMOSEXUALITY SCALE
A. P. MacDonald, Jr.

Address
Director
Univesity of Wisconsin System-wide Center for the Study of
Minorities and the Disadvantaged
Office of the Graduate School
P.O. Box 413
The University of Wisconsin-Milwaukee
Milwaukee, WI 53201

Available From
Publications Office
Center for the Study of Human Sexuality
4105 Medical Parkway, Suite 205
Austin, TX 78756

General Description
A self-report scale measuring subject's attitudes toward homosexuality regardless of their own sexual orientation. Three forms are available: General (Form G), Lesbian (Form L), and Male (Form M).

Subjects
Intended for use with widely divergent populations, though currently used with college students and faculty.

Mode of Rating
Self-report.

Items
28 items with 9-scale positions for each item. Example: "Homosexuals should not be permitted to raise children."

Scoring
Each item is responded to by the subject on a 9-point scale from "strongly agree" to "strongly disagree." The resulting score is the total score for all items.

Reliability

A study of 94 male and 103 female undergraduates at West Virginia University yielded the following alpha coefficients: Form M = .94, Form L = .93. Another study of 47 male and 57 female students and faculty at WVU using Form G yielded an alpha coefficient of .93. One hundred eighty-eight male students at Iowa State University were given a 22-item form, using 5-point rather than 9-point scales and yielded split-half reliability of .93.

Validity

Information of validity is available from the references.

References

MacDonald AP, Jr, Games RG: Some characteristics of those who hold positive and negative attitudes toward homosexuals. *J Homosex 1* :9, 1974.

MacDonald AP, Jr, Huggins J, Young S, Swanson RA: Attitudes toward homosexuality: Preservation of sex morality of the double standard? *J Consult Clin Psychol 40*:161, 1973.

Nash JE: Reactions to homosexuals: Effects of sex-role attitudes and similarity on attraction. Master's thesis, Iowa State University, 1977. (Ms. Janet E. Nash, 205A Old Botany, Psychology Department, Iowa State University, Ames, IA 50010.)

SEMANTIC DIFFERENTIAL AS MEASURE OF SEXUAL ATTITUDES
I. M. Marks and N. H. Sartorius

First Author's Address

Institute of Psychiatry
The Maudsley Hospital
Denmark Hill
London S.E.5, England

Available From

First author.

General Description

This is a scale devised for assessing attitudinal change during treatment for sexual deviation.

Subject

Adults.

Mode of Rating

Self-report.

Items

20 sexual and nonsexual concepts (i.e., call girl, flirt, my father) rated on 13 bipolar semantic differential scales (i.e., pleasant-unpleasant, repulsive-seductive, bad-good). Factor analysis revealed three dimensions: general evaluation, sex evaluation, and anxiety. The scale detected significant attitudinal changes in the general evaluation and sex evaluation dimensions but not in the anxiety dimension during the treatment of 8 patients with sexual deviations.

Reliability
The scale showed adequate stability on test-retest within 24 hours.

Validity
It was found useful in the follow-up of sexual deviants over 2 years after treatment. It has also been employed for the assessment of progress during treatment and follow up of patients with sexual dysfunction.

References
Marks IM: in *Behavioral Psychotherapy for Neurosis,* Published by Royal College of Nursing, London, 1977.
Marks IM, Gelder MG, Bancroft J: Sexual deviants two years after electric aversion. *Br J Psychiatry 117*:173, 1970.
Marks IM, Sartorius NH: A contribution to the measurement of sexual attitude in sexual deviations. *J Nerv Ment Dis 154*:441, 1968.

CALIFORNIA MARRIAGE READINESS EVALUATION
M. P. Manson

Address
Western Psychological Services
12031 Wilshire Boulevard
Los Angeles, CA 90025

Available From
Address above.

General Description
Designed to provide help to the counselor by identifying areas of potential maladjustment and conflict. The eight areas assessed are character structure, emotional maturity, marriage readiness, family experiences, dealing with money, planning ability, marriage motivation, and compatibility.

Subjects
Premarital couples.

Mode of Rating
Self-report.

Items
115 true-and-false questions.

Reliability and Validity
No information available.

Reference
Harper RA: In OK Buros (Ed), *The Seventh Mental Measurement Yearbook,* Highland Park, NJ, Gryphon Press, 1972. (A critical evaluation included.)

MOSHER FORCED-CHOICE GUILT INVENTORY (FCGI)
D. L. Mosher

Address
Department of Psychology
University of Connecticut
Storrs, CONN 06268

Available From
Author.

General Description
The FCGI consists of pairs of answers to a series of incomplete sentence stems. On each item the subject is to select which of the two answers best applies to him/her. The FCGI was developed and is scored to reveal three separate aspects of guilt: sex guilt (SG), hostility guilt (HG), and morality conscience (MC). The author views the instrument as measuring the personality disposition of guilt rather than the feeling state.

Subjects
Adults.

Items
Male and female versions of the test, with the male version consisting of 150 items and the female version 78 items.

Mode of Rating
Self-report.

Reliability
The author reports high levels of both internal consistency and test-retest reliability in reference publications.

Validity
Multitrait-multimethod studies have shown good convergent and discriminant validity for the scale; confirmatory factor analysis has provided support for validation of the construct dimensions of guilt.

References
Mosher DL: Measurement of guilt in females by self-report inventories. *J Consult Clin Psychol 32*:690, 1968.
Mosher DL: Sex differences, sex experience, sex guilt and explicit sexual films. *J Soc Issues 29*:95, 1973.
Mosher DL: The meaning and measurement of guilt. In CE Izard, JL Singer (Eds), *Emotions and Personality in Psychopathology*. New York, Plenum Press, 1978.

A SEX ATTITUDE SURVEY AND PROFILE
G. McHugh and T. G. McHugh

Address
Family Life Publications, Inc.
P.O. Box 427
Saluda, NC 28773

Available From
Above address.

General Description
This instrument is in process of development and is currently published in a preliminary edition. Its aim is to register individual responses to stated attitudes, beliefs and values concerning a wide variety of sexual feelings, activities and practices.

Subjects
Adults.

Mode of Rating
Self-report.

Items
107 statements to which the individuals indicate their degree of agreement or disagreement by circling the appropriate response (five choices from "strongly agree" to "strongly disagree"). Sample item: "Couples who want to have a successful sex partnership should tell each other about all past sex experiences."

Reliability and Validity
No information available.

Reference
None available.

SEX KNOWLEDGE INVENTORIES (SKI)
G. McHugh

Address
Family Life Publications, Inc.
P.O. Box 427
Saluda, NC 28773

Available From
Address above.

General Description
The inventories are designed to assess individual levels of sex knowledge. There are two tests labeled Forms X and Y.

Subjects
The SKI Form X (Revised 1968) is aimed for adults (college level and above). The SKI Form Y is primarily aimed at youth groups and for sex education classes at the high school level. It has been developed for use as a basic teaching tool and has not been revised since its first complete edition in 1955.

Mode of Rating
Self-report.

Items
Form X—80 multiple-choice questions that take approximately 30 minutes to complete. The test set includes a test booklet, answer sheets, a scoring key, and a marriage counselor's manual. This manual provides detailed discussions of the best answers for each question.

Form Y—100-item questionnaire and a scoring key. High school and college norms are available.

Reliability and Validity
No information available.

Reference
Buros OK (Ed): *The Seventh Mental Measurement Yearbook,* Highland Park, NJ, Gryphon Press, 1972. (A review of SKI included.)

SEXUAL ANXIETY SCALE
M. Obler

Address
Department of Educational Services
Brooklyn College
Brooklyn, NY 11210

Available From
Author. Also on microfilm at The New School for Social Research Library, 65 Fifth Avenue, New York, NY 10003.

General Description
The Sexual Anxiety Scale measures cognitively experienced social and sexual anxieties. The content of the items range from anxiety experienced during contact with a member of the opposite sex to intravaginal penetration.

Subjects
Adults.

Mode of Rating
Self-report.

Items
22 items in separate forms for males and females.

Reliability
Author reports a .92 reliability coefficient.

Validity
Author reports a .62 validity coefficient with intensity of sexual dysfunction.

Reference
Obler M: Systematic desensitization in sexual disorders. *J Behav Ther Exp Psychiatry 4*:93, 1973.

AN INVENTORY OF MARITAL CONFLICTS
D. H. Olson and R. G. Ryder

First Author's Address
32–28 Birchtree Lane
Silver Springs, MD 20906

Available From
First author.

General Description
The aim of this inventory is to obtain interaction data on conflict resolution and decision-making process in couples. The instrument consists of vignettes which describe various types of marital conflicts that are usually relevant to couples. Responses to four specific questions are requested in relation to each item: (1) "Who is primarily responsible for the problem?" (2) a content question that suggests a way for resolving the problem which couples can accept or reject; (3) "Have you had a similar problem?" and (4) "Have you known other couples who have had similar problems?" After the couple individually responds to these questions on separate forms, they are brought together with the instruction of fully discussing each conflict situation and jointly decide (1) "Who is primarily responsible for the disagreement, the husband or the wife?" and (2) "Which of two mutually exclusive ways of resolving the conflict is best?" The couple is encouraged to limit the interaction to a 30-minute period while the discussion is tape recorded. The authors indicate that this instrument may be used for research and diagnostic purposes and may also be of value to evaluate process change resulting from treatment.

Subjects
Couples.

Mode of Rating
Two types of data are obtained: the first is derived from the individual or joint response forms and the second is obtained from the tape-recorded discussion of the cases by the couple. The discussion is coded on 29 categories in an interaction coding system which has been developed to measure objectively the interaction process, and it is analyzed by a computer.

Items
18 vignettes divided into 12 conflict items and 6 nonconflict items.

Reliability and Validity
The authors provide data on internal consistency of "win scores" based on 200 couples. They also provide information on instrument validity.

Reference
Olson DH, and Ryder RG: *Inventory of Marital Conflicts (IMC): An experimental interaction procedure. J Marr Fam 32:443, 1970.*

SEXUAL RESPONSE PROFILE
R. J. Pion

Address
Department of Obstetrics/Gynecology
Kapiolani Hospital

1319 Punahov Street
Honolulu, Hawaii 96814

Available From
Enabling Systems, Inc.
444 Hoborn Lane
Honolulu, Hawaii 96815

General Description
The questionnaire covers knowledge, attitudes, past and present practices in sexual areas. The items were chosen via an analysis of suggested questions offered by a sample of physicians seeing couples with sexual and marital problems. It is reported as useful to pinpoint problem areas related to the patient's sexual history.

Subjects
Individuals and couples presenting with sexual dysfunctions.

Mode of Rating
Self-administered.

Items
80 items. Each item is scored according to the content of the subject and the scores, therefore, range from yes/no response, through checkmarks to scaled items. There is no overall scoring system for the entire inventory.

Reliability
None published.

Validity
Face validity only.

Reference
Annon JS. *The Behavioral Treatment of Sexual Problems.* Vol 2, *Intensive Therapy.* Honolulu, Enabling Systems, 1976.

PATIENT PROFILE
R. J. Pion

Address
Department of Obstetrics/Gynecology
Kapiolani Hospital
1319 Punahov Street
Honolulu, Hawaii 96814

Available From
Enabling Systems, Inc.
444 Hobron Lane
Honolulu, Hawaii 96815

General Description
A questionnaire for female patients covering general medical history, gynecological history, contraceptive history, and reproductive plans. Further items allow the patient to

indicate the areas where help is required, e.g., sexual satisfaction, knowledge, etc. It is useful to indicate those patients requiring medical help and the areas where problems exist.

Subjects
Female patients only.

Mode of Rating
Self-administered.

Items
Specific questions in each of the areas of general medical, gynecological, and contraceptive history and reproductive plans.

Scoring
Direct response. No scores.

Reliability
None published.

Validity
Face validity only.

Reference
Annon JS: *The Behavioral Treatment of Sexual Problems.* Vol 2, *Intensive Therapy.* Honolulu, Enabling Systems, 1976.

REISS PREMARITAL SEXUAL PERMISSIVENESS SCALES
I. L. Reiss

Address
Department of Sociology
University of Minnesota
Minneapolis, MINN 55455

Available From
Reiss IL, *The Social Context of Premarital Sexual Permissiveness.* New York, Holt, Rinehart and Winston, 1967.

General Description
This attitudinal scale is concerned with acceptance of three categories of premarital physical acts: kissing, petting, and coitus. Each behavior is considered in the context of different conditions of affection. Conditions of affection are divided into four categories: engagement, love, strong affection, and no affection. Each of the three physical conditions is qualified by each of the four affection-related states, making a total of 12 statements which the respondent is asked to agree or disagree with either "strongly," "moderately," or "slightly."

Subjects
This scale has been frequently used on populations from 16 years and up as an indicator of premarital sexual attitudes.

Mode of Rating
Self-report.

Items
12 items. Sample item: "I believe that petting is acceptable for the male when he is in love." In order to prevent ambiguity, key terms used in the scales, such as love, petting, and strong affection, are defined. A respondent can be rated in two ways: (1) how he responds to the scale statements of his own sex and (2) how he responds to scale statements using the opposite sex as the referent.

Reliability and Validity
Systematic evaluation shows that the scale meets the requirements of Guttman scaling. Evidence of reliability and validity of the scale has been provided by the author and by independent investigators.

References
Hampe GD, Ruppel HJ: The measurement of premarital sexual permissiveness: A comparison of two Guttman scales. *J Marr Fam 36*:451, 1974.
Reiss IL: *The Social Context of Premarital Sexual Permissiveness.* New York. Holt, Rinchart and Winston, 1967.
Reiss IL, Miller L: A theoretical analysis of heterosexual permissiveness. University of Minnesota, Family Study Center, Technical Bulletin, No. 2, 1974.

HETEROSEXUAL BEHAVIOR INVENTORIES
C. H. Robinson and J. S. Annon

Address
Enabling Systems, Inc.
444 Hobron Lane
Honolulu, Hawaii 96815

Available From
Address above.

General Description
A checklist form to assess range and frequency of an individual's heterosexual behavior repertoire. The statements include solitary as well as partner-directed behaviors. There are female and male forms available. Each consists of items paralleling the items in the Heterosexual Attitude Scales. It offers an effective method for ascertaining the heterosexual behavior repertoire of the patient.

Subjects
Patients presenting with sexual dysfunctions.

Mode of Rating
Self-administered.

Items
77 items including self-observation and observation of a partner, interpersonal sexual behaviors, and a wide range of direct sexual behavior. Frequency of engaging in a particu-

lar behavior is indicated at the "0" "1 to 3 times," "4 to 10 times," "11 or more times," and "regular basis" levels.

Reliability
None published.

Validity
Face validity only.

Reference
Annon JS: *The Behavioral Treatment of Sexual Problems.* Vol 2, *Intensive Therapy.* Honolulu, Enabling Systems, 1976.

HETEROSEXUAL ATTITUDE INVENTORIES
C. H. Robinson and J. S. Annon

Address
Enabling Systems, Inc.
444 Hobron Lane
Honolulu, Hawaii 96815

Available From
Address above.

General Description
(See *Heterosexual Behavior Inventories.*) A self-administered checklist to assess patient's attitudes toward specifically sexually related activities and experiences. The 77 items chosen are identical with those of the Heterosexual Behavior Inventories. The range of scoring is a 7 level scale from Dislike (very much, much, some, neither like or dislike) to Like (some, much, to very much). Clinically the inventory is able to pinpoint sexual activities eliciting positive or negative attitudes. The comments for the Heterosexual Behavior Inventories apply equally to this inventory. Both inventories have an added dimension when each partner's response is compared.

SEX ATTITUDE SCALE
G. Rotter

Address
Educational Foundation for Human Sexuality
Montclair State College
Upper Montclair, NJ 07043

Available From
Author.

General Description
An attitude scale concerning a variety of sexual issues such as sex roles, sex education, sexual intercourse, marital relationships, etc. The items are to be rated on a Likert scale of

seven degrees of agreement, from totally agree to totally disagree. From an initial population of over 1200 sex-attitude statements, four scale forms were developed, each containing 198 attitudinal items and only 5 of which appeared on all forms.

Items

100 items. Samples: "An increase in premarital sex is desirable"; "Teenagers know less about sex than they realize"; "Having money helps the love relationship"; "Sex is perfectly valid without a couple being in love."

Scoring

Items are scored on a 7-point scale from +3 to −3 indicating agreement or disagreement with the statement. Statistical analysis revealed two basic sexually adjusted types and two sexually maladjusted types. The author identifies these prototypes as the "Banacek" and "Marcus Welby" and their antithesis, "Archie Bunker" and "Woody Allen." Means for the four types are presented for each item as well as means for a college student sample by sex (male and female).

Reliability

Not reported.

Validity

In one study a number of items achieved statistical significance from raters' assignment into sexually adjusted and maladjusted categories.

References

Rotter GS: Clinician perspectives of adjusted and maladjusted sex attitudes. Unpublished manuscript available from the author.

Rotter GS: Genital and socio-sexual attitudes of college students. Paper presented at the Eastern Psychological Association, Washington, DC, 1973.

THE MALE IMPOTENCE TEST
A. El Senoussi

Address

Western Psychological Services
12031 Wilshire Boulevard
Los Angeles, CA 90025

Available From

Address above.

General Description

The author claims that the test is capable of discriminating between psychogenically impotent men, organically impotent men and nonimpotent individuals. It is a questionnaire from which five scores are devised: (1) reaction to female rejection, (2) flight from male role, (3) reaction to male inadequacy, (4) an organic factor, and (5) total score.

Subjects

Adult males.

Mode of Rating
Self-report.

Reliability and Validity
No data is provided on reliability. The validity of the test as a diagnostic instrument has been criticized by Ellis (1972). A recent study failed to show that this test was of value in the differential diagnosis of organic versus psychogenic impotence (Beutler et al. 1975).

References
Beutler LE, et al: MMPI and MIT discriminators of biogenic and psychogenic impotence. *J Consult Clin Psychol 43*:899, 1975.
Ellis A: The Male Impotence Test. In OK Buros (Ed), *The Seventh Mental Measurement Yearbook*. Highland Park, NJ, Gryphon Press, 1972.

SEXUAL DEVELOPMENTAL SCALE FOR FEMALES
A. El Senoussi

Address
Western Psychological Services
12031 Wilshire Boulevard
Los Angeles, CA 90025

Available From
Address above.

General Description
The scale attempts to measure the "relative degree of sexual frigidity" and to identify aspects or causative factors involved.

Subjects
Adult females.

Mode of Rating
Self-report.

Items
177 items with seven factor scores: lack of feminine identity, free-floating anxiety, unpleasant sexual encounter, passive sex aversion, flight into sex, sexual insufficiency, and early negative conditioning.

Reliability
Limited to total scores.

Validity
None available.

Reference
Ellis A: In OK Buros (Ed), *The Seventh Mental Measurement Yearbook*. Highland Park, NJ, Gryphon Press, 1972. (A critical examination included.)

SEX QUESTIONNAIRE FOR COLLEGE STUDENTS
R. Shipley

Address
Health Sciences Department
William Patterson College of New Jersey
Wayne, NJ 07470

Available From
Address above.

General Description
This questionnaire covers such areas as information and attitudes toward contraception, physiology and anatomy, sex-role behaviors, marriage, and child rearing. In addition, there are questions pertaining to the personal characteristics of the responder.

Subjects
College students.

Mode of Rating
Self-report.

Items
156 true-false items, multiple-choice items, and Likert Scale.

Reliability
Author reports an internal consistency reliability coefficient of .74.

Validity
No information available.

References
None available.

CARING RELATIONSHIP INVENTORY
E. L. Shostrom

Address
Educational and Industrial Testing Service
P.O. Box 7234
San Diego, CA 92107

Available From
Address above.

General Description
This instrument has been designed to provide a measure of the "essential elements of love or caring in human relationships." Development of the inventory was based on responses of criterion groups: successfully married couples, troubled couples in counseling, and divorced individuals. Five elements of love are measured by independent scales: affec-

tion, friendship, eros, empathy and self-love, plus two scales based on concepts of being loved and deficiency love. Two forms of the inventory are used: one for the male rating the female and one for the female rating the male.

Subjects
Couples.

Mode of Rating
Self-report.

Items
83 items to which the examinee responds either true or false, first as applied to the other member of the couple (spouse, fiance, etc.) and second as applied to his "ideal."

Reliability
Data on split-half reliability and intercorrelation values among the scales is provided in the test manual.

Validity
No information available.

Reference
Ellis A. In OK Buros (Ed), *The Seventh Mental Measurement Yearbook.* Highland Park, NJ, Gryphon Press, 1972. (A critical examination included.)

DYADIC ADJUSTMENT SCALE
G. B. Spanier

Address
Division of Individual and Family Studies
and Department of Sociology
Pennsylvania State University
University Park, PA 16802

Available From
Spanier GB: Measuring dyadic adjustment: New scales for assessing the quality of marriage and similar dyads. *J Marr Fam 38*:15, 1976.

General Description
This scale is aimed at assessing the quality of marriage and other similar dyads. It is based on four empirically verified components of dyadic adjustment which can be used as subscales: dyadic satisfaction, dyadic cohesion, dyadic consensus, and affectional expression.

Subjects
Couples.

Mode of Rating
Self-report.

Items

32 items, most of which are scored on 6-point scales. Individuals specifically interested in assessing dyadic satisfaction may use a 10-item subscale for this purpose.

Reliability

Total scale reliability is .96. Data is also provided by the author indicating that the four scale components also have high reliability.

Validity

Evidence is presented by the author suggesting content, criterion-related and construct validity.

Reference

Spanier GB, Cole CL: Toward clarification and investigation of marital adjustment. *Int J Soc Fam* 6:121, 1976.

ATTITUDE TOWARD WOMEN SCALE
J. T. Spence and R. Helmreich

First Author's Address
Department of Psychology
University of Texas
Austin, TX 78712

Available From
Selected Documents in Psychology
American Psychological Association
1200 Seventeenth Street, NW
Washington, DC 20036

General Description
A self-report scale bearing on the vocational, educational, social and intellectual roles of women, including their freedom and independence, interpersonal relationships, and sexual behavior.

Subjects
Females or males.

Mode of Rating
Self-report.

Items
55 items consisting of a declarative statement for which there are four response alternatives: agree strongly, agree mildly, disagree mildly, and disagree strongly. Examples: "It is alright for wives to have an occasional, casual, extramarital affair"; "Husbands and wives should be equal partners in planning the family budget." The items cover attitudes toward the economic, intellectual, social, and interpersonal capabilities of women as well as women in comparison with men.

Scoring

Each item is given a score from 0 to 3, with 0 representing choice of the response reflecting the most traditional, conservative attitude and 3 the most liberal, profeminist attitude. Each subject's score is obtained by summing the values for the individual items according to the scoring key identifying the most conservative choice. Separate machine scorable answer sheets are available. The 55 items have been descriptively categorized into six more or less independent content groups: I. Vocational, educational and intellectual roles (17 items); II. Freedom and independence (4 items); III. Dating, courtship, and etiquette (7 items); IV. Drinking, swearing and dirty jokes (3 items); V. Sexual behavior (7 items); and VI. Marital relationships and obligations (17 items).

Validity

Normative data has been collected on two samples of 754 female and 710 male introductory psychology students and 298 mothers and 232 fathers of these students. Significant differences between the sexes regardless of age were found on 47 of the 55 items. The data were analyzed for interrelationship of the items. Factor loadings correlated in many cases to the categories listed in the general description. A study of 343 female and 267 male students given the AWS and the California Personality Inventory Feminity Scale showed no correlation between liberalness of attitudes to women and dubious "femininity" or heterosexuality in women nor between antifeminism and masculinity in men. Use of the scale in a pre-post study of outcome of group sex therapy with women revealed changes in five items in the expected direction reflecting increased sexual and economic equality in relationships but no changes in the overall score.

References

Spence JT, Helmrich R: Who likes competent women? Competence, sex-role, congruence of interests and subject's attitudes toward women as determinants of interpersonal attraction. *J Appl Soc Psychol,* July-Sept, 1972a.

Spence JT, Helmreich R: A test of our times: A comparison of university students and their parents on the attitudes toward women scale. Unpublished manuscript, 1972b.

Spence JT, Helmreich R: The attitudes toward women scale: An objective instrument to measure attitudes toward the rights and roles of women in contemporary society. Special Document, American Psychological Association.

MAFERR INVENTORY OF MASCULINE AND FEMININE VALUES
A. Steinman and J. Fox

First Author's Address

Maferr Foundation, Inc.
124 East 28th Street
New York, NY 10016

Available From

Address above.

General Description

There are two distinct inventories in the series; one oriented toward feminine values, the other oriented toward masculine values. Five forms of each of the two basic inventories exist, designed to measure male and female sex-role perceptions, both of themselves and of each other. The first author began work on the scales in the 1950s and has been utilizing them ever since.

Subjects
Adult males and females.

Mode of Rating
Self-report.

Items
34 items in each scale expressing value judgments with which the subject agrees or disagrees on 5-point Likert scales.

Reliability
Author reports a split-half coefficient of .80.

Validity
Author cites over 15 studies in a revised manual published in 1979.

References
Steinman AG, Fox DJ: Maferr Inventories of Feminine (MIFV) and Masculine (MIMV) Values, 1979. This manual and a complete bibliography are available from above.

THE SEX INVENTORY
F. C. Thorne

Address
Brandon, VT 05733

Available From
Clinical Psychology Publishing Company
Brandon, VT 05733

General Description
This is an empirically developed inventory comprising nine scales designated as follows: Factor A. Sex Drive and Interest; B. Sexual Maladjustment and Frustration; C. Neurotic Conflict Associated with Sex; D. Sexual Fixation and Cathexes; E. Repression of Sexuality; F. Loss of Sex Controls; G. Homosexuality; H. Sex-Role Confidence; and I. Promiscuity. This instrument has been used in the study of sexual attitudes and behavior of adult men in several normal and clinical groups. The self-report inventory may be supplemented by interview and observational verification. The instrument is intended to measure "state" phenomena which may be in constant flux or change.

Subjects
Adult males.

Mode of Rating
Self-report.

Items
200 questions requiring a true or false answer.

Reliability and Validity
Data are available on test-retest reliability of scale scores and on the factorial characteristics of the instrument.

References

Allen RM, Haupt TD: The Sex Inventory; Test-retest reliabilities of scale scores and items. *J Clin Psychol 22*:375, 1966.

Thorne FC: A factorial study of sexuality in adult males. *J Clin Psychol 22*:378, 1966b.

Thorne FC: The Sex Inventory. *J Clin Psychol 22*:367, 1966a.

Thorne FC: A grand research design for measuring psychological states. *J Clin Psychol 32*:209, 1976a.

Thorne FC: A new approach to psychopathology. *J Clin Psychol 32*:751, 1976b.

Thorne FC, Haupt TD: The objective measurement of sex attitude and behavior in adult males. *J Clin Psychol 22*:395, 1966.

SEXUAL ATTITUDES AND BELIEFS INVENTORY
D. Wallace

Address

Human Sexuality Program
University of California Medical School
350 Parnassus Avenue, Suite 700
San Francisco, CA 94143

Available From
Address above.

General Description
The inventory is a scale oriented to the attitudes and information about sexual behavior of the reporting individual. In addition, information concerning sexual experience is elicited. Anatomy and physiology, contraception, sexual behavior, psychosexual development, variations, disorders, laws, and populations are major content headings.

Subjects
Normal adults.

Mode of Rating
Self-report.

Items
250 items: true-false items and Likert scales.

Reliability
Author reports test-retest coefficients between .75 and .85 with a 4-week separation on a population of medical students.

Validity
No information available.

References
None available at present.

SEX EXPERIENCE SCALES FOR MALES AND FEMALES
M. Zuckerman

Address
Department of Psychology
University of Delaware
Newark, DEL 19711

Available From
Address above.

General Description
This instrument consists of a list of sexual behaviors people have engaged in from the most basic (e.g., kissing, etc.) to various coital positions and oral-genital contact. These are two scales: one for males and one for females. They have been arranged in a hierarchy from most endorsed to least endorsed by the population on whom they were developed. Since they are Guttman scales, they possess the characteristic that the endorsement of a scale item usually means that the individual has experienced all items before it.

Subjects
Both scales were developed on college undergraduates.

Mode of Rating
Self-report.

Items
12 items requiring forced choice responses of whether or not the subject has had that experience.

Reliability
Coefficients of reproducibility and rank-order correlations between males and females are provided in the reference article.

Reference
Zuckerman M: Scales of sex experience for males and females. *J Consult Clin Psychol* *41*:27, 1973.

SEX QUESTIONNAIRE
M. Zuckerman

Address
Department of Psychology
University of Delaware
Newark, DEL 19711

Available From
Address above.

General Description
The questionnaire is a scale designed to provide an evaluation of sexual attitudes and behaviors. It is comprised of 10 subscales which vary in length from several 1-item scales to the Heterosexual Experience Scale of 14 items.

Subjects
Adult normals.

Mode of Rating
Self-report.

Items
91 items rated along 5-point scales. The instrument is composed of the following subscales: heterosexual experience, attitudes toward heterosexual behavior, parental attitudes, homosexual experience, orgasmic experience, masturbatory experience, number of heterosexual partners, and desire to view erotic movies.

Reliability
Test-retest reliabilities on four samples are presented in the reference below.

Validity
None available.

Reference
Zuckerman M, Tushup R, Finner F: Sexual attitudes and experience: Attitude and personality correlates and changes produced by a course in human sexuality. *J Consult Clin Psychol 44*:7, 1976.

Summary of Scale Characteristics

First Author Relevant Reference	Name of Instrument	Referent Population				Rater			Objective of Instrument	Type of Data Collected	Reliability	Validity
		Normals	Pt. With Sex. Dysf.	Heterosex. Couples	Other	Self	Signif. Other	Profes.				
Abramson, PR et al J Consult & Clin Psych 43:485, 1975	Negative Attitudes toward Masturbation Scale	x	x			x			Assessment of attitudes, false beliefs & affects associated with masturbation	Inventory consisting of 30 items which are rated on a 5-pt. Likert Scale	x	x
Annon, J Behavioral Treatment of Sexual Problems, Vol. 2, Honolulu	Sexual Pleasure Inventory	x				x			Inventory of people, objects & Behaviors that are pleasurable	130 items - 5 possible responses to each item		
Annon, J Behavioral Treatment of Sexual Problems, Vol. 2, Honolulu	Sexual Fear Inventory	x				x			Inventory of people, objects & behaviors that lead to fear	130 items - 5 possible responses to each item		
Barrett-Lennard, GT Dept. of Human Relations U of Waterloo, Ontario Canada	Relationship Inventory			x		x	x	x	Measurement of 4 dimensions of interpersonal relationships	64 items rated on a 6-pt. scale. Several forms available	x	x
Bem, S J Consult & Clin Psychol 42:155, 1974	BEM Sex Role Inventory	x				x			Characterization of a person along two independent masculine & feminine dimensions	60 masculine, feminine & neutral personality characteristics rated on a 7-pt. scale	x	x
Bentler, PM Behavioral Research 6:21, 1968 & 6:27, 1968	Heterosexual Behavior Assessments	x	x			x			Assessment of the range of heterosexual experiences	Questionnaire with 21 classes of heterosexual behaviors arranged in hierarchical manner		
Bienvenu, MT Family Co-ordinator 19:26, 1970	Marital Communication Inventory			x					Assessment of degree of awareness in marital communication	46 items rated on 4-pt. scales		
Bodin, AM, Comrey, AL et al (Eds), A Source Book for Mental Health Measures, Los Angeles: Human Interaction Research Inst., 1973, p.187	Self Disclosure Questionnaire			x		x	x		Assessment of self-disclosure to spouse & of perceived disclosure from the spouse on various aspects of living	Questionnaire with 52 items scored on an 8-pt. scale		
Derogatis, LR: Psychological Assessment of the Sexual Disabilities. In J. Meyer (Ed) Clinical Management of the Sexual Disorders, Balt.: Wms. & Wilkins, 1976	Derogatis Sexual Functioning Inventory (DSFI)	x	x			x	x		The measurement of 8 domains of sexual functioning plus measures of psychological symptoms & affect	245 items measured on a variety of distinct scales felt to be relevant to adequate sexual functioning	x	x
Feldman, M et al Behavioral Research & Therapy 4:289, 1966	The Sexual Orientation Method				x	x			Assessment of relative degree of homo- & hetero-orientation of men who show homosexual behavior	Questionnaire in a semantic differential format with 120 pairs of items concerning attitudes toward men & women	x	x
Foster, AL J Clin & Consulting Psychol. In Press	Sexual Compatibility Test			x		x			Assessment of the sexual relationship of couples	101 behaviors measured on 6 scales with 37 multiple choice items		
Frenken, J Sexuality Experience Scales. Amsterdam: Swet Sand Zeitlinger. In press	Sexuality Experience Scales (SES)	x	x			x			Assessment of various aspects of sexual behavior and experience	83 multi-formatted questions	x	x

Summary of Scale Characteristics—*Continued*

First Author Relevant Reference	Name of Instrument	Normals	Pt. with Sex. Dysf.	Heterosex. Couples	Other	Self	Signif. Other	Profess.	Objective of Instrument	Type of Data Collected	Reliability	Validity
Fretz, B Perceptual & Motor Skills 22:201, 1966	Sex Attitude Questionnaire	x	x			x			Measures attitude toward behaviors and situations broadly construed as sexual in our society	12 concepts, each evaluated on 7 bipolar dimensions	x	x
Greene, BL A Clinical Approach to Marital Problems. C Thomas, Pub., 1970	Biographical Marital Questionnaire			x		x	x		Gathering background data about couple, & information on affectional aspects of marriage, divisions of responsibility, areas of difficulty, etc.	22 open-ended questions to be completed independently by each partner		
Gurland, BJ et al Arch Gen Psych 27:259,	The Structured & Scale Interview to Assess Maladjustment (SSIAM)				x			x	Measurement of maladjustment in five life areas	11 dimensions for each life area scored on a 10-pt. scale	x	x
Harbison, JJM et al Arch Sex Behav 3:357, 1974	A Questionnaire Measure of Sexual Interest	x	x			x			Measurement of degree of interest in various sexual situations	140 items - subject marks the adjectival statement that best describes his/her response to the sexual situation in question	x	x
Hollender, MH Arch Gen Psych 20:188, 1969	Body Contact Questionnaire	x	x			x			Assessment of desire for body contact	12 questions scored on a 5-pt. Likert Scale	x	
Hoon, EF et al Arch Sex Behav 5:291, 1976	Sexual Arousability Inventory	x	x			x			Assessment of female sexual arousability	28 descriptions of sex activities. Respondent rates, each on the basis of how sexually arousing the activity is to her	x	x
Hudson, WW Unpublished manuscript	Index of Marital Satisfaction			x		x			Measures degree of dissatisfaction with the interpersonal component of the couple's relationship	25 items rated on 5-pt. scales		
Hudson, WW Univ. of Hawaii, School of Social Work, 1976	Index of Sexual Satisfaction			x		x			Measures degree of dissatisfaction with the sexual component of the couple's relationship	25 items rated on 5-pt. scales		
Kahn, N Family Proc. 9:449, 1970	Marital Communication Scale			x		x			A situational measure of non-verbal communication accuracy	16 items	x	x
Kurtz, R J Clin Psychol 26:149,1970	Body Attitude Scale	x	x	x	x				Measures global attitudes towards the outward form of a person's body	30 body concepts rated on semantic differential scales	x	x
Lawlis, FG Various dissertations See text	The Four Relationship Factor Questionnaire	x	x	x	x				Identifies perceptions of people's relationships in a wide range of interaction	44 items rated on a 4-pt. scale	x	x
Lief, HL et al Ctr. for Study of Sex Ed in Med, 405 Chestnut St., Phila.	Sex Knowledge & Attitude Test	x							Assessment of sexual attitudes, knowledge & experience	149 multiple choice items	x	x
Locke, H et al Marriage & Family Living 21:251, 1959	Lock-Wallace Marriage Inventory			x		x	x		Assessment of marital adjustment	15 to 27 questions asking husbands & wives how they perceive or assess their marriage	x	x
LoPiccolo, J et al Arch Sex Behav 3:585, 1974	Sexual Interaction Inventory			x		x	x		Assessment of sexual adjust. ment & sexual satisfaction	Ratings on questions related to 17 items covering a range of heterosexual behaviors	x	x

Summary of Scale Characteristics—*Continued*

First Author Relevant Reference	Name of Instrument	Normals	Pt. with Dys.	Sexes	Couples	Other	Self	Signif. Other	Profess.	Objective of Instrument	Type of Data Collected	Reliability	Validity
MacDonald, AP Jr. J of Homosex 1:9, 1974	Sex-Role Survey	x					x			Measures subject's attitudes towards sex-roles	53 items scored along 9-pt. scales of agreement	x	x
MacDonald, AP Jr. J Consult Clin Psychol 40:161, 1973	Attitudes toward Homosexuality Scale	x					x			Measures subject's attitudes toward homosexuality	28 items rated on 9-pt. scales	x	x
Marks, IM et al J of Nerv Ment Disease 145:441, 1968	Semantic Differential as a Measure of Sexual Attitude			x			x			Assessment of attitudinal changes toward sex	20 sexual & non-sexual concepts rated on 13 bipolar semantic differential scales	x	x
Manson, MP Western Psychological Services	California Marriage Readiness Evaluation				x		x	x		Identification of areas of probable maladjustment or conflict with premarital couples	115 true & false questions		
Mosher, DL J Cons & Clin Psych 32:690, 1968	Forced-Choice Guilt Inventory	x	x				x			Assessment of 3 aspects of guilt	Forced-Choice to incomplete stems	x	x
McHugh G et al Family Life Pub., Inc.	Sex Attitude Survey and Profile	x					x			Records individual responses to attitudes and values concerning sexual feelings, activities and practices	107 items rated on a 5-pt. scale		
McHugh, G Family Life Pub., Inc.	Sex Knowledge Inventories	x					x			Assesses individual levels of sex knowledge	80 multiple choice questions		
Obler, M J Beh. Ther & Exp Psych 4:93, 1973	Sexual Anxiety Scale	x	x				x			Measures cognitively experienced social and sexual anxieties	22 items	x	x
Olson, DH et al J Marriage & Family	Inventory of Marital Conflicts				x		x	x		Gathering of interaction data on conflict resolution & decision making	Independent & joint responses to 18 vignettes which describe various types of marital conflicts	x	x
Pion, J Behavioral Treatment of Sexual Problems Vol. 2, Honolulu	Sexual Response Profile	x					x			Sexual knowledge & attitudes	80 items		
Pion, J Behavioral Treatment of Sexual Problems Vol. 2, Honolulu	Patient Profile					x	x			Questionnaire for female patients covering general medical & gynecological history, contraception & reproductions	Direct response to questions. No scores		
Reiss, IL The Social Context of Premarital Sexual Permissiveness, NY: Holt, Rinehart & Winston, 1967	Reiss Premarital Sexual Permissiveness Scales	x					x			Assessment of attitudes concerning acceptance of 3 categories of premarital sexual	12 items with 6 possible choices, rated for self & opposite sex	x	x
Robinson, CH et al Behavioral Treatment of Sexual Problems, Vol. 2 Honolulu	Heterosexual Behavior Inventory	x	x	x			x			Attitude & emotional response to sexually related activities	77 items		
Rotter, G Unpublished manuscript	Sex Attitude Scale	x	x				x			Attitude scale concerning a variety of sexual issues	100 items scored on a 7-pt. scale		

Summary of Scale Characteristics—*Continued*

First Author / Relevant Reference	Name of Instrument	Normals	Pt. with Sex. Dysf.	Heterosex. Couples	Other	Self	Signif. Other	Profess.	Objective of Instrument	Type of Data Collected	Reliability	Validity
El Senoussi, AE The Male Impotence Test Western Psychological Services, LA, Ca, 1964	The Male Impotence Test		x			x			Discrimination between psychologically impotent men, organically impotent & non-impotent individuals	Questionnaire		
El Senoussi, A West. Psychol. Serv.	Sexual Development Scale for Females	x	x			x			Distinction between "frigid" & "non-frigid" women	177 questions, 38 scores, 7 factors		
Shipley, R Wm. Paterson College of NY, 300 Pompton Rd., Wayne, NJ	Sex Questionnaire for College Students	x				x			Inventory of attitudes, knowledge & behavior in a wide range of sex-related fields	156 items of varying formats		
Shostrom, EL Educ. & Indust. Testing Service	Caring Relationship Inventory	x	x	x		x	x		Assessment of 7 types of love nurturing, peer, romantic, altruistic, self, being & exploitative	83 true-false items	x	
Spanier, GB J of Marriage & the Family 38:15, 1976	Dyadic Adjustment Scale			x		x			Assessment of empirically determined components of dyadic adjustment	32 items, most of which are scored on a 6-pt. scale	x	x
Spence, JT et al American Psychological Association	Attitudes toward Women Scale	x				x			Assessment of women's roles including interpersonal relationships and sexual behavior	55 items consisting of a statement for which there are 4 response alternatives		x
Steinmann, A Maferr Foundation, Inc. 174 E. 28th St., NYC	Maferr Inventories of Masculine & Feminine Values	x				x			Assessment of female & male sex role perceptions, both of themselves & of each other	34 statements of male & female activities & satisfactions rated on a 5-pt. scale	x	x
Thorne, FC J Clin Psych 22:367, 1966	The Sex Inventory	x			x	x			"Assessment of sexual interests, drives, attitudes, adjustment, conflict, cathexes, controls & sociopathic tendencies"	200 questions requiring true or false answers	x	x
Wallace, D Human Sex Program, U of CA Med School, SF, CA 94143	Sexual Attitudes & Beliefs Inventory	x				x			Assessment of sexual attitudes, knowledge & range of sexual experience	250 items. True-false and Likert Scales	x	
Zuckerman, M J Consult Clin Psychol 41:27, 1973	Sex Experience Scales for Males & Females	x				x			Assessment of Sexual Behaviors people have engaged in	12 items requiring force choice responses	x	
Zuckerman, M J Consult Clin Psych 44:7, 1976	Sex Questionnaire	x				x			Assessment of sexual attitudes & experiences	91 multiple choice items	x	

Journal of Sex & Marital Therapy
Vol. 5, No. 3, Fall 1979

Assessing Sexual Behavior in Couples

Joseph K. Nowinski, PhD, and Joseph LoPiccolo, PhD

ABSTRACT: The role of formal assessment in the practice of sex therapy with couples is discussed. A case is made for the use of behaviorally oriented paper-and-pencil tests of the self-report variety, in clinical settings, at two points in time: prior to any therapist-client contact and following completion of therapy. Such procedures are both efficient and effective, yielding information relevant to diagnosis, treatment planning, and development of clinical skills. Assessment procedures used routinely at the Stony Brook Sex Therapy Center are described and illustrated using sample cases. The authors suggest that behavioral assessment approaches have considerable clinical potential which has yet to be fully realized.

This article will describe the clinical assessment of couples as it is practiced at the Sex Therapy Center of the Department of Psychiatry and Behavioral Science, School of Medicine, State University of New York at Stony Brook. It is our hope that this presentation not only will serve to illustrate clinical assessment of sexual behavior, but also will encourage clinicians to consider the use of formal assessment procedures as an adjunct to couples therapy.

The Stony Brook Center is an active research clinic, and, as such, it utilizes a variety of standardized as well as experimental self-report tests of the paper-and-pencil variety to evaluate comparatively different approaches to the treatment of sexual dysfunction. However, research is not the only use for our assessment data, and in this paper we will attempt to show how the tests we use provide us with information which plays a central role in the actual conduct of our clinical practice.

It is our impression that the use of standardized assessment procedures for clinical (as opposed to research) purposes has fallen increasingly into disfavor, or at least disuse, in recent years. In clinical psychology training

Dr. Nowinski is a Post-Doctoral Fellow and Dr. LoPiccolo is Professor of Psychiatry in the Department of Psychiatry and Behavioral Science, State University of New York at Stony Brook. Please address requests for reprints to Dr. Joseph LoPiccolo, Professor of Psychiatry, Department of Psychiatry and Behavioral Science, Health Sciences Center, State University of New York at Stony Brook, Stony Brook, New York 11794.

Writing of this paper was supported in part by Grant #MH1462103 (NIMH).

programs, for instance, psychological testing as an area of study has been de-emphasized or eliminated in many cases. In many others the prevailing attitude seems to be that assessment is a skill which may be obligatory to the curriculum but which is of highly questionable utility. The development and/or standard use of assessment procedures in clinical practice settings is seldom encouraged; rather, courses in clinical assessment tend to focus more or less exclusively on critical reviews of the literature. With such attitudes prevailing it is not surprising that assessment fails to find its way into clinical practice.

Originally, the trend away from clinical assessment may not have been entirely unfounded. Research evidence accumulating over the past 20 years or more has been at best equivocal with respect to the predictive utility of classical psychological testing. Particular targets have included such traditional instruments as the Rorschach, Thematic Apperception Test, and the Minnesota Multiphasic Personality Inventory—in short, tests of the projective and empirical varieties. Viewed from this perspective, the gradual loss of interest in traditional psychological assessment procedures paralleled the decline of the medical-intrapsychic view as the prevalent model of human behavior favored by academic psychologists. Meanwhile, the ascendance of behaviorism has brought with it new concepts of behavior, pathology, and treatment. The behavioral model calls for an approach to assessment which is based on a different set of assumptions from those underlying either projective or empirical tests. Rotter,[1] in articulating the behavioral approach to personality assessment, emphasized such principles as the use of test referents that closely approximate the criterion and the careful specification of the criterion situation. These principles contrast sharply with those characterizing projective and empirical measures. Thus, if one wishes to know about clients' sexual functioning, one asks questions about sex rather than inferring sexual functioning from responses to ambiguous, non-sex-relevant test stimuli, as for example ink blots. Measures such as the Sexual Interaction Inventory,[2] which seeks to predict sexual functioning by asking questions whose content references specific sexual behaviors and situations, illustrates the application of behavioral principles to test construction. It differs significantly from projective and empirical measures. Readers who are interested in pursuing the issue of behavioral personality assessment are referred to Rotter[1] and to a more recent article by Goldfried and Sprafkin,[3] for further discussion of these theoretical issues is beyond the scope of this paper.

Recent years have witnessed a burgeoning in the field of behavioral personality assessment. During this span of time many behaviorally oriented measures of demonstrated predictive utility have appeared in the literature. Despite its availability, however, this technology does not seem to have become popular in clinical settings. There may be several reasons for this, the first being the relative recency of the technology itself. Many practicing clinicians may be unaware of the existence of tests which they might potentially find useful. Another reason may have to do with the essentially negative attitude toward clinical work and testing that too often characterizes training programs. A third reason would seem to lie in clinicians' stereotypical attitudes toward behavioral measures. Usually such tests are seen as "research" instruments, suitable perhaps for nomothetic investigations and sensitive to group differences but having little applicability to the task of designing helpful treatment procedures for a particular client with specific problems. We feel that this attitude is inaccurate; behavioral assessment can be of great value to the practicing clinician. We would like to demonstrate here how such tests *can* be used productively in a strictly clinical context. Clinics large and small, which do not regard themselves as research centers, as well as the solo private practitioner may equally benefit, in our opinion, from judicious application of carefully selected paper-and-pencil assessment of the behavioral type. In contrast to being a useless expenditure of time and money, and/or an imposition on the client, such procedures can help make clinical practice both more effective and efficient, and are thus in the best interest of the client.

PROCEDURE FOR ASSESSING SEXUAL BEHAVIOR IN COUPLES

In order for assessment to be useful, it must be *specifically* relevant to the task at hand. That is, the connection between test content, diagnostic schema, and treatment strategy must be direct and simple. If one is doing sex therapy with couples, therefore, one would want to collect data that focuses in on the *relationship* between two people, and more specifically on the *sexual aspect* of that relationship. If properly selected and collected early enough, information obtained from standard tests may be of great value to the therapist in correctly diagnosing the nature of the problem and selecting a viable treatment strategy from among the various options available. In addition, it can be helpful in anticipating resistances and in proferring an honest prognosis and treatment contract to the prospective clients. These are, in fact, precisely the clinical purposes to which we put our standard assessment package at the Stony Brook Center.

Couples seen for treatment at the Sex Therapy Center are asked to fill out batteries of questionnaires at several points in time. Specifically, it is our practice to ask each partner to complete a standard battery on five occasions: prior to being seen for an initial (intake) interview; just prior to starting therapy (usually 6 to 8 weeks after intake); immediately following completion of therapy; 3 months after treatment ends; and 1 year post-treatment. This schedule allows for efficient diagnostic evaluation, documents "spontaneous remission" as opposed to therapy-induced change, and permits evaluation of the maintenance (or relapse) of therapeutic effects. The batteries are mailed to the clients, who fill out the questionnaires in the privacy of their homes and then mail them back to the center in prepaid envelopes.

Such extensive testing procedures as the above may be of questionable utility in a strictly clinical setting. One might justifiably argue, for instance, that testing for spontaneous remission is a moot issue for the practicing clinician. Similarly, one might argue against repeated follow-up procedures as unnecessarily costly, given their yield to the clinician. Although this might mitigate against having as many as two long-term follow-up assessments after completion of therapy, we would argue that the data gathered from at least one such delayed follow-up is highly valuable and well worth the time required to gather, score, and interpret it. As clinicians, we should all be invested in documenting the lasting effectiveness of our procedures. In regard to skill and time required to gather, score, and interpret test data, the former two functions may be efficiently accomplished by clerical personnel; they require less time than might be expected. Interpretation is, of course, best done by the clinician who, after all, is the person who stands to gain from the information. We find that routine follow-up provides data which lead to a general sharpening of diagnostic and treatment skills. It also reflects, on a concrete level, our interest in our clients. It is our experience that clients respond quite positively to this interest, that they take it as a sign of professionalism, and that they do not feel burdened by it.

THE ASSESSMENT BATTERY

The measures which comprise the standard assessment battery currently in use at the Stony Brook Center are described below. Clinical application of these tests, using sample cases, will be illustrated in a later section.

General Information Form

The General Information Form (GIF) has evolved from the work of the center over a period of several years. It asks standard, interviewlike questions to obtain basic data such as absolute frequencies of sexual contact, masturbation, duration of foreplay and intercourse, frequency of erectile failure, orgasm, and so on. As such it is useful in orienting the clinician and in providing a tentative diagnosis. The GIF also inquires into the couple's usual pattern of sexual interaction as well as their relative satisfaction with this pattern. Normative data has been gathered from 164 nondysfunctional couples and provides useful standards for purposes of comparison. From the GIF one may form initial impressions regarding likely areas of dyadic conflict and tentatively assess the compatibility and reasonableness of each partner's sexual goals. Some clinicians may choose to share some GIF data, and most especially normative data, with their clients toward the end of educating a couple who may hold unrealistic expectations. Others prefer merely to note the existence of incompatibilities or unrealistic goals and to pursue them at later points in the treatment.

Locke-Wallace Marriage Inventory

The Locke-Wallace Marriage Inventory,[4] or LWMI, is a global measure of marital satisfaction. At the Sex Therapy Center we use the Kimmel and Van der Veen[5] revision of this scale, which uses weighted scores. The LWMI yields a total score for each partner that reflects their degree of satisfaction with the relationship. Both total scores and partner discrepancies in total scores have been found to be predictive of the viability of a relationship.[6] The means for males and females respectively on this instrument are 110 ($SD = 16$) and 108 ($SD = 16$). Scores below 90, therefore, indicate a generally disturbed relationship. The utility of this test at the center, then, is that it gives us some sense of the overall stability of a relationship and the amount of conflict within it. In some cases we prefer to refer a couple for marital as opposed to sex therapy, or else to contract with them to work on manageable marital problems concurrently in sex therapy, since it is our experience that severe conflict mitigates against success in treatment of a specific sexual dysfunction. Although the LWMI is but one piece of data that would enter into such a decision, it is an important one which is available early.

On a more microscopic level, clients' responses to certain LWMI items seem to be particularly significant vis-à-vis prognosis, especially their reply to questions such as "Have you ever wished you had not married?" and "If you had your life to live over again, would you marry the same person, marry a different person, or not marry at all?" Finally, part of the LWMI is a problem checklist which gives the clinician a convenient summary of each partner's perceptions of areas of dyadic conflict. We frequently find this list is useful in drawing tentative treatment plans.

Sexual Interaction Inventory

The Sexual Interaction Inventory (SII) focuses on 17 specific sexual activities (see Table 1). It asks each member of a client couple for a variety of information relative to each of these activities, including how much they enjoy it and their estimate of their partner's enjoyment of it.

Development of the SII has been previously reported,[2] and the interested reader may refer to this literature for additional information relative to its internal statistical characteristics and validity. Suffice it to

TABLE 1
Sexual Interaction Inventory Item List

Item	Description
A	The male seeing the female when she is nude.
B	The female seeing the male when he is nude.
C	The male and female kissing for one minute continuously.
D	The male giving the female a body massage, not touching her breasts or genitals.
E	The female giving the male a body massage, not touching his genitals.
F	The male caressing the female's breasts with his hands.
G	The male caressing the female's breasts with his mouth (lips or tongue).
H	The male caressing the female's genitals with his hands.
I	The male caressing the female's genitals with his hands until she reaches orgasm (climax).
J	The female caressing the male's genitals with her hands.
K	The female caressing the male's genitals with her hands until he ejaculates (has a climax).
L	The male caressing the female's genitals with his mouth (lips or tongue).
M	The male caressing the female's genitals with his mouth until she reaches orgasm (climax).
N	The female caressing the male's genitals with her mouth (lips or tongue).
O	The female caressing the male's genitals with her mouth until he ejaculates (has a climax).
P	The male and female having intercourse.
Q	The male and female having intercourse with both of them having an orgasm (climax).

say that the instrument differentiates dysfunctional from nondysfunctional couples and that it is sensitive to treatment effects. The SII can be scored conveniently by hand in approximately 10 minutes and requires no special training. A simple calculator can reduce even this modest investment of time. For those who have access to computer facilities a program is available that will yield additional data not discussed here.*

*For information about copies of this program, which is written in FORTRAN IV, write to Dr. J. LoPiccolo, Health Sciences Center, State University of New York of Stony Brook, Stony Brook, New York 11794.

Manual scoring nets 11 raw scores, which are then easily converted to standard scores and charted to produce a visible profile. Each SII scale has a mean of 50 and a standard deviation of 10. Scoring has been arranged so that higher scale scores indicate greater pathology (conflict, dissatisfaction, etc.), with scores above 70 indicating a large degree of pathology. The SII may also be interpreted more microscopically, as for example when the clinician wishes to look for congruence versus discordance of partners' attitudes toward specific behaviors. The 11 SII clinical scales, and their respective meanings, are described below.

Scale 1: Frequency dissatisfaction—male.   In this scale actual frequencies of occurrence of the various sexual activities included in the SII, as reported by the male partner, are compared to the frequencies with which he says he would like these activities to occur. Scale 1 is thus an index of the male partner's relative dissatisfaction with the current repertoire of sexual behaviors he and his partner are engaging in. It may be taken to reflect the strength of his motivation for change in the sexual sphere of the relationship. High scores indicate a generalized dissatisfaction, but they do not reveal the *direction* of desired change (i.e. increased versus decreased frequency). To ascertain the latter one must look at the pattern of specific responses. While high Scale 1 scores usually indicate a desire for more frequent activity, it is sometimes the case that a high Scale 1 score is constructed partly of desires to see some activities increase in frequency and others decrease in frequency. Similarly, perusal of discreet responses in an otherwise low Scale 1 score may reveal a strong desire on the part of the male to see one or two behaviors occur more or less frequently. Depending upon the female partner's responses to these same items, such responses may provide important clues as to areas of conflict and likelihood of change. In some cases of elevated Scale 1 scores the female partner may be discovered to be very inhibited or even to find sex aversive. It may also happen, however, that both partners are merely sexually naive, shy to experiment, or unable to communicate effectively. Finally, high Scale 1 scores may indicate a general loss of interest in sex on the part of the female partner.

Scale 2: Self-acceptance—male.   Scale 2 compares the male partner's current level of enjoyment to his desired level of enjoyment of each sexual act listed in the SII. When these two differ across many items, a high score, indicating generalized frustration, will result. A low Scale 2 score, however, may camouflage dissatisfaction in one or two delimited areas so that perusal of real-ideal discrepancies relative to specific sexual behaviors is often clinically useful. Such isolated discrepancies may reflect idiosyncratic inhibitions that are a source of discomfort for the client. In general, high Scale 2 scores should lead one to inquire further into the male partner's self-image as well as his current level of self-esteem. Very likely both of these will be found to be lacking. Very low Scale 2 scores may indicate low motivation for treatment or a reflection of the male's view that he is sexually very competent. Such men tend to place the responsibility for sexual problems entirely on their partner and can as a result be difficult clients.

Scale 3: Pleasure mean—male.   Unlike Scale 2, which compares actual to desired levels of pleasure, Scale 3 is simply the male client's average level of self-reported enjoyment of all 17 activities comprising the SII. A high pleasure mean indicates sexual anhedonia, but, in and of itself, it may not suggest motivation to change as clearly as Scales 1 and 2 do. Low pleasure ratings for specific sexual acts may be taken as reflecting personal tastes. Relative dislike of specific activities may or may not be indicative of dyadic conflict, depending on the partner's frequency dissatisfaction scores for those activities. A very high pleasure mean indicates a definite need for inquiry toward the end of discerning etiology. This may range from general depression to loss of interest in the partner, active aversion (disgust, fear, etc.), and sexual orientation conflict.

Scale 4: Perceptual accuracy—male of female.   This scale shows how accurately the male perceives his partner's sexual preferences. Specifically, it compares *his* responses to the question "I think my mate finds this activity . . ." to *her* self-reported enjoyment of that activity, then sums these discrepancies (when they exist) across all 17 SII items. High Scale 4 scores suggest poor dyadic communication, which may then become a treatment goal. Poor sexual communication, in turn, may be attributable to the male partner, in that he is either not vigilant for or else misperceives his partner's communications. Alternatively, the female partner may be either reticent to communicate or ignorant of how to do so. More commonly, both partners need help in establishing effective communication. It is also possible for one partner to perceive the other accurately while he or she is not accurately perceived. In this case the therapist's communications goals become somewhat more circumscribed.

Scale 5: Mate acceptance—male of female.   Scale 5 compares the way the male currently perceives his partner's enjoyment of sexual activities to the reaction of his fantasized "ideal" sexual partner. That is, his estimates of how much his partner enjoys an activity are compared to how much he would like her to enjoy it. If his perceptual accuracy (Scale 4) is good, then a high Scale 5 score indicates that the man is dissatisfied with his partner's actual responses and, specifically, that she does not enjoy things as much as he would like her to. She may be inhibited in general, or she may be adverse to specific types of activities, for example, oral-genital contact. Frequently these same activities do not occur as often as the man would like, and elevations of Scale 5 are, therefore, often associated with elevations of Scale 1. The female partner may be expected to resist her partner's press for more frequent occurrence of these activities that she dislikes but he wants. The therapeutic goal may then be some form of compromise, greater acceptance on the part of the man of his partner's sexual tastes, or enhancement of her ability to enjoy various sexual activities.

When perceptual accuracy by the male is poor, high Scale 5 scores must be viewed with caution. It may be that the man is underestimating his partner's enjoyment. If this is so, ineffective communication must be suspected and tentatively identified as a treatment goal. On the other hand, it sometimes happens that the male partner is actually *overestimating* the woman's pleasure, yet is still dissatisfied with it. Such cases obviously present a more trying clinical challenge, since improved communication will generally exacerbate the conflict.

Microscopic analysis of mate acceptance scores often points to isolated areas of concern that may be fruitful foci for therapeutic intervention.

Scale 6: Total disagreement. As a global index of sexual satisfaction, representing totals drawn across Scales 1, 2, 4, 5, 7, 8, 10, and 11, Scale 6 is the best single index of the extent of sexual conflict and dissatisfaction in the relationship. In general, the higher the Scale 6 score, the more difficult and time-consuming should the therapist expect the case to be. A treatment contract based on extremely brief or minimal therapist-client contact may be contraindicated when Scale 6 is very high.

(*Note:* Scales 7 through 11 are simply the female counterparts of Scales 1 through 5 and hence will be described more briefly.)

Scale 7: Frequency dissatisfaction—female. Scale 7 is analogous to Scale 1 but applies to the female rather than the male partner. Interpretation of Scale 7, therefore, is analogous to interpretation of Scale 1. A high Scale 7 score clearly indicates dissatisfaction, but one must again consult the pattern of responses to all 17 SII items in order to be sure of the direction of motivation, i.e., toward lesser or greater frequency. A generalized desire for more frequent occurrence of all behaviors is commonly associated with premature ejaculation and erectile failure. It is also found in couples in which the male partner is inhibited or adverse to sexual contact. On occasion, both partners may be sexually naive and/or inhibited, and one or both may be desirous of change. This will be reflected in Scales 1 and 7. If both are elevated, one may infer that both partners are motivated to change their sexual repertoire. Closer analysis of their response patterns will then reveal whether or not their desired changes are compatible. This will, in turn, be significant for prognosis and treatment planning. When only one of Scales 1 and 7 is elevated or when their underlying motivations are discordant, dyadic conflict and client resistance may be expected, and treatment will usually take more time.

Scale 8: Self-acceptance—female. Scale 8 is analogous to Scale 2 but refers to the female partner. High Scale 8 and Scale 2 scores alike suggest low self-esteem in regard to sexual responsiveness. Not infrequently they are associated with some depression. Scale 8 elevation is a frequent concomitant of orgasmic dysfunction. Configurally, when Scale 8 (or Scale 2) is elevated but Scale 7 (or Scale 1) is not, the individual is in effect saying that she (or he) is satisfied with the existing sexual repertoire in terms of frequency but is not enjoying it as much as she would like. Conversely, elevations in Scale 7 (or Scale 1), when associated with a Scale 8 (or Scale 2) score in the normal range, indicate enjoyment of sexual activity but dissatisfaction with the repertoire. Finally, elevations in both Scales 7 and 8 (or 1 and 2) suggest extensive dissatisfaction both with the relationship and one's self. All of these combinations are associated with client motivation, but of different kinds (i.e., toward different ends); as such, they bear important implications for treatment planning.

Scale 9: Pleasure mean—female.   Analogously to Scale 3, Scale 9 reflects the female partner's self-reported enjoyment of sex, averaged over the 17 SII items. By itself Scale 9 is not as good an index of the female client's motivations as are Scales 7 and 8. Extremely high scores indicate a need for inquiry and elaboration. They may reflect depression, sexual aversion, anxiety, dyadic conflict, or sexual orientation conflict.

Scale 10: Perceptual accuracy—female.   Scale 10 tells how accurately the female perceives her partner's sexual tastes and preferences. High scores, meaning poor perceptual accuracy, may be attributable to either or both partners. Unless there is strong evidence to the effect that the male partner is communicating effectively but is being purposefully ignored, sexual communication training is indicated.

Scale 11: Mate acceptance—female of male.   Scale 11 provides the clinician with an indication of the extent to which the female partner perceives her male partner's sexual responses as ideal. It is analogous to Scale 5. If the perceptual accuracy (Scales 4 and 10) of both partners is good, then Scales 5 and 11 may be taken as an index of sexual/compatibility. If both Scales 5 and 11 are low (indicating that the partner's self-reported responses to each sexual act is congruent with what her or his partner would like them to be), one may infer that the sexual relationship is complementary. Such a condition is not, of course, incompatible with a sexual dysfunction, which may have an etiology not at all related to dyadic factors. As it concerns treatment of that dysfunction, however, compatibility in the sexual relationship generally speaks well for the prognosis of the case.

In the event that perceptual accuracy of one or both partners is poor, the aforementioned compatibility may, of course, be based in sheer fantasy or even dissimulation. A real estimate of compatibility would in such cases have to follow improved sexual communication.

Marriage and Sex Defensiveness Scales

Obviously, when assessment is based on paper-and-pencil, self-report inventories, the question of clients' truthfulness in responding becomes a real issue. In an effort to test for dissimulation in test taking, development of a Marriage Defensiveness Scale (MDS) and a Sex Defensiveness Scale (SDS) was supported by the Sex Therapy Center.[7] Unlike global measures of defensiveness these scales focus specifically on marital and marital-like relationships and seek to measure the extent to which partners are motivated to "fake good" when responding to questions that inquire into their relationship in general and their sexual relationship in particular. As such, the defensiveness scales may be used much like their analogue on the MMPI—the "Lie" Scale—which is to shed light on the probable validity of other test scores. High defensiveness scores render validity of other assessment data (and especially the LWMI and SII) more or less questionable. One's best move under such circumstances is to assume that pathology is somewhat understated by the test scores themselves. Moreover, high defensiveness scores in one or both partners should lead the clinician to anticipate a defensive posture toward therapy in general, manifested in a resistance to confrontation.

The male MDS consists of 32 items. The mean MDS score for 164 nondysfunctional men is 11 ($SD = 8$). The female MDS has 37 items; the mean is 13 ($SD = 8$).

The male SDS contains 16 items and has a mean of 6 ($SD = 6$). The female SDS has 15 items and has a mean of 6 ($SD = 4$).

CLINICAL USE OF THE ASSESSMENT BATTERY

In this section we will extend the foregoing discussion of clinical assessment by analyzing two sample cases. In each case we will attempt to make conservative inferences based on data available *prior to* any therapist-client contact. Hopefully, such modeling will be of use to the reader who wishes to experiment with the sort of clinical assessment we are describing here. The cases we have chosen for presentation are not atypical, in terms of the extent of personal and dyadic conflict they present, for those applying for treatment at the Sex Therapy Center. In assessing each of them, we will proceed in the order in which the various assessment devices were described earlier, which is the sequence used by the majority of our clinicians.

Sample Case: Mr. and Mrs. A

Contact with the Stony Brook Sex Therapy Center was made by Mrs. A, age 38. According to information obtained over the telephone, she and her husband, age 46, had been married for 18 years. It was the first marriage for her, the second for him. They had five children who ranged in age from 5 to 16. Shortly after the birth of the youngest child Mrs. A voluntarily underwent a tubal ligation, a procedure her husband reportedly opposed.

The As both had high school educations. Mr. A was employed as a skilled laborer, while Mrs. A worked part time in a semiskilled capacity. According to her, Mr. A had been unable to obtain more than a partial erection, insufficient for penetration, for approximately 3 years. That is, the last sexual experience which included intercourse had occurred 3 years earlier. For the previous year and a half Mr. A had experienced erectile difficulties with increasing frequency. At the time of Mrs. A's call neither partner had initiated any sexual contact whatsoever for approximately 18 months. During this time, however, Mr. A had consulted with two physicians, the second a urologist, who could find no organic basis for his difficulty. Based on these findings the urologist referred the As to the Center.

Assessment data. The As responses to the General Information Form (GIF) appear in Table 2. Their responses (center columns) may be compared to the median responses of 164 nondysfunctional couples (right-hand column). It can be seen that both partners confirm the sexual abstinence initially reported by Mrs. A. Moreover, each claims not to masturbate at all, suggesting a total absence of sexual outlet for both.

Since the As had not attempted any sexual contact in over a year, their responses relative to duration of foreplay and intercourse may be considered minimally relevant at

TABLE 2
General Information Form
Sample Case A

Question	Male Response	Female Response	Median Response
Frequency of intercourse	Not at all	Not at all	Twice a week
Desired frequency of intercourse	Once a week	Once a week	3 or 4 times a week
Usual initiator	I always do	Mate usually	I usually do
Desired Initiator	Myself usually	Mate and I equally often	Mate and I equally often
Frequency of masturbation	Not at all	Not at all	Once a month
Years of intercourse with mate	More than 10 years	More than 10 years	7 to 10 years
Duration of foreplay	11 to 15 minutes	16 to 30 minutes	11 to 15 minutes
Duration of intercourse	7 to 10 minutes	11 to 15 minutes	4 to 7 minutes
Your feelings about sex with mate	Extremely satisfactory	Extremely satisfactory	Moderately satisfactory
Mate's feelings about sex with you	Extremely satisfactory	Extremely satisfactory	Moderately satisfactory
Response to sex advances by mate	Accept reluctantly	Usually accept with pleasure	Usually accept with pleasure
Orgasm through masturbation	Never	Have never tried	Nearly always, 90% of the time
Orgasm through carressing by mate	Have never tried	Nearly always, 90% of the time	Always, 90% of the time
Orgasm through intercourse	Have never tried	Nearly always, 90% of the time	Nearly always, 90% of the time
Reaction to Pronography	Somewhat aroused	Greatly aroused	Somewhat aroused
Erectile problems before intercourse	Never	Never	Never
Erectile problems during intercourse	Nearly always, 90% of the time	Nearly always, 90% of the time	Never

the present time, except perhaps to note that the duration of their sexual encounters in the past exceeds that generally reported. It may appear ironic that, given their circumstances, both partners rate their feelings about sex as extremely satisfactory. On the one hand, one might take this as evidence of defensiveness. However, it may also be that the As were reporting their *past* feelings about sex together. The last piece of data provided by the GIF is an extremely important one, since it casts additional light on the nature of the dysfunction, at least as it existed as of a year and a half prior to Mrs. A's call to the center. Both partners agree that Mr. A's erectile failure was specifically associated with coitus. It appears that he was regularly able to achieve an erection during foreplay but that he would then lose the erection once intercourse was attempted. This mitigates against the hypothesis of organic etiology and tentatively narrows the expected goal of treatment from achieving and maintaining erections to maintaining erections.

On the Locke-Wallace Marriage Inventory (LWMI) Mr. A scored 118, Mrs. A 111. According to Kimmel and Van der Veen's norms, then, the As report that their relationship is generally quite satisfactory. Perusing individual LWMI items revealed that both partners said they rarely wished they had not married and that they would both marry the same partner had they their lives to live over again. In addition, of 21 specific problem areas listed in the LWMI, Mr. A cites three as having been salient at one time or another in his marriage; they are money, sex, and ill health. Mrs. A cites only one problem area, that being sex.

The As' Sexual Interaction Inventory (SII) appears in Table 3. From it several clinical hypotheses may be drawn. First, Mr. A's score on Scale 1 indicates that he is *not* particularly dissatisfied with the couple's (presumably past) typical sexual repertoire, whereas Mrs. A's comparable score on Scale 7 suggests that she has been dissatisfied with it. Analysis of individual item responses brings this discrepancy into clearer focus, revealing that Mrs. A would like more nongenital sexual contact (SII items A. B. D, and E), while Mr. A is reportedly content with a varied but somewhat genitally focused sexuality.

Both partners seem to be accepting of their own level of sexual responsiveness (Scales 2 and 8). It may be inferred, therefore, that neither could be expected to feel a strong desire to change their preferences and, further, that Mr. A may resist his wife's desire for change in the sexual repertoire. Mr. A, on the other hand, does acknowledge a significant loss of sexual enjoyment per se (Scale 3), presumably due to his erectile problems.

The shared lack of perceptual accuracy which characterizes the As' relationship (Scales 4 and 10) is suggestive of poor sexual communication. While the precise etiology of this communications deficit is not revealed by these data, its existence is noted. Based on these scales alone, sexual communication may be anticipated to be a problem area within the relationship and a likely target for therapeutic intervention. The fact that the couple has apparently avoided sexual contact for over a year, however, might serve to forewarn the therapist that improved communications might not be easily achieved.

The two partner acceptance scores (Scales 5 and 11) may be interpreted at their face value, i.e., that the relationship is sexually compatible. The couple's poor perceptual accuracy, however, again must be considered, along with the alternative hypothesis that shared misconceptions plus a desire to avoid confrontation might be responsible for these scores. Lastly, the couple's total disagreement score (Scale 6) is only moderately elevated and would, in and of itself, suggest a good prognosis.

The final piece of data available to the therapist prior to meeting with the As comes from their scores on the Sex and Marriage Defensiveness scales. For Mr. A these were 12 and 15, respectively; for Mrs. A they were 10 and 11. As compared to the norms presented earlier, only the SDS scores may be considered high. In short, it would seem that both partners are straightforward with respect to their overall relationship but that they are motivated to present an exaggeratedly favorable impression of their sexual relationship. Based on these data they would be expected to minimize the severity and breadth of any sexual malaise, a fact the clinician would do well to keep in mind. In addition, one might predict that both partners would react with anxiety if and when the issue of sexual conflict is broached and, further, that they may well unite to resist the prospective therapist in her or his efforts to uncover and work with such conflict.

In sum, the preintake assessment battery defines the sexual problem as centered in Mr.

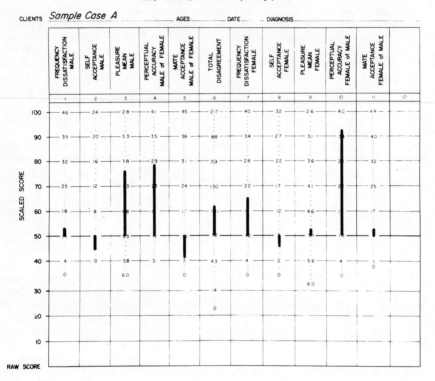

TABLE 3
SEXUAL INTERACTION INVENTORY
Joseph LoPiccolo, Ph.D. and Jeffrey C. Steger, Ph.D.

A. who appears to suffer from secondary erectile failure which is typified by a pattern of loss of erection on coitus. Evidently, then, Mr. A can experience sexual arousal, but he loses that arousal when intercourse begins. Mrs. A does not appear to be dysfunctional, having a history of being able to achieve orgasm through manual and oral stimulation as well as during intercourse. It further appears that, as a couple, the As have a long-standing pattern of avoidance of conflict and communication. This pattern may be most pronounced in the sexual sphere of the relationship, where both partners seem highly motivated to present the situation in a positive light and to minimize the extent and degree of any sexual disharmony. Mr. A acknowledges a loss of sexual satisfaction and ostensibly wishes to restart the sexual relationship; otherwise he appears to be essentially satisfied with himself and with the sexual repertoire which typified the relationship in the past. Mrs. A, on the other hand, seems more dissatisfied with the relationship and may be expected to desire change, privately if not publicly. While both she and her husband claim to be satisfied with each other as sexual partners, this satisfaction may be based on misconceptions or fantasy more than real knowledge. Overall, the therapist may expect to encounter resistance from both partners to confronting potential problem areas and from Mr. A with respect to the issue of changing the repertoire which characterized the sexual relationship in the past.

All of the above represent clinical hypotheses drawn from assessment data that have been collected prior to any client-therapist contact. They must of course be viewed with caution. At best they are tentative formulations that require validation through face-to-face contact. They are, however, highly useful in that they prepare the therapist and serve as guidelines which can facilitate the actual therapeutic process considerably.

Sample Case: Mr. and Mrs. B

Mr. and Mrs. B, age 47 and 35 respectively, were married for 8 years and had two young children at the time they applied for treatment. In this case it was Mr. B who telephoned the clinic, presenting two complaints, both centered in his wife. The first was that she was primary inorgasmic (preorgasmic); the second was that she disliked being touched on her breasts or genitals by him during sexual contact. While this was Mrs. B's first marriage, Mr. B had been married before. Both held graduate degrees. Mr. B worked as a teacher, while Mrs. B devoted her time exclusively to housekeeping and child rearing.

Assessment data. The GIF (Table 4) for the Bs confirms that Mrs. B indeed believes that she has never experienced an orgasm via any means of stimulation. Because she also reports that she has never attempted masturbation, one might hypothesize tentatively that she is inhibited with respect to self-pleasuring. Together, the Bs' responses to the GIF also offer limited support to the second of Mr. B's complaints: Mrs. B apparently accepts her husband's sexual advances with reluctance, and he perceives this attitude on her part. One might wonder, given these circumstances, why they engage in intercourse as often as they do and whether Mrs. B may be submissive, her husband coercive, or both. In any case, the sheer fact that the Bs engage in intercourse daily, while Mrs. B would prefer that it occurred once a week, would lead one to suspect that she is at the very least unhappy with the present situation.

According to the GIF, Mr. B has a level of sexual interest somewhat in excess of that reported by most men. This is reflected in a total sexual outlet of more than seven orgasms per week, a frequency he is apparently happy with. He evidently experiences erectile failure during intercourse on occasion, but he would not be described as dysfunctional.

On the LWMI Mr. and Mrs. B scored 84 and 80, respectively. These scores are approximately two standard deviations below the mean and are indicative of considerable dyadic disharmony. Specific areas of conflict cited by Mr. B include religion, amusements, and sex. He indicated, however, that he would remarry the same woman. Mrs. B cites religion, amusements, choice of friends, selfishness, child rearing, and gambling as specific areas of conflict. Moreover, she indicated that she would marry a different sort of man had she to do it over again. In sum, sexual difficulties would seem to be but one facet of a generally troubled relationship here, and the prospective therapist should anticipate the possibility of either having to work in several areas concurrently (thereby extending the treatment contract), of prescribing concurrent marital and sex therapy, or even of postponing sex therapy until such time as other dyadic issues are resolved.

The B's SII profile appears in Table 5, where one is struck first of all by the sheer number of highly elevated scales. Both partners report that they are unhappy with the frequency with which various sexual activities occur. Closer inspection, however, reveals somewhat discrepant goals. Mr. B would like virtually all behaviors to occur more often, whereas his wife would like some to occur more often, others less often. Specifically, she reportedly wants sexual activities B, D, E, G, I, and L (Table 1) to happen more often than they do. Activities F, H, J, K, N, O, and P, on the other hand, are occurring more often than Mrs. B would prefer. The Bs, then, are motivated toward making changes in their sexual repertoire, but the direction of their motivations are conflicting rather than syntonic. A clear pattern seems to be emerging wherein Mrs. B feels put upon by her husband's sexual demands.

Comparing self-acceptance scores and pleasure means suggests that Mr. B is the more personally secure of the two, at least insofar as his sexual self-image is concerned. He enjoys sex (Scale 3) and feels satisfied with his level of sexual response (Scale 2). Mrs. B, in

TABLE 4
General Information Form
Sample Case B

Question	Male Response	Female Response	Median Response
Frequency of intercourse	Once a day	Once a day	Twice a week
Desired frequency of intercourse	Once a day	Once a week	3 or 4 times a week
Usual initiator	I usually do	Mate always	I usually do
Desired initiator	Mate and I equally often	Mate and I equally often	Mate and I equally often
Frequency of masturbation	Once every two weeks	Not at all	Once a month
Years of interaction with mate	More than 10 years	More than 10 years	7 to 10 years
Duration of foreplay	1 to 3 minutes	11 to 15 minutes	11 to 15 minutes
Duration of intercourse	7 to 10 minutes	11 to 15 minutes	4 to 7 minutes
Your feelings about sex with mate	Slightly satisfactory	Slightly satisfactory	Moderately satisfactory
Mate's feelings about sex with you	Extremely unsatisfactory	Moderately satisfactory	Moderately satisfactory
Response to sex advances by mate	Usually accept with pleasure	Accept reluctantly	Usually accept with pleasure
Orgasm through masturbation	Nearly always, 90% of the time	Have never tried	Nearly always, 90% of the time
Orgasm through carressing by mate	Never	Never	Always, 90% of the time
Orgasm through intercourse	Nearly always, 90% of the time	Never	Nearly always, 90% of the time
Reaction to pronography	Somewhat aroused	Not aroused	Somewhat aroused
Erection problems before intercourse	Never	Never	Never
Erection problems during intercourse	Seldom, 25% of the time	Never	Never

contrast, neither enjoys sex (Scale 9) nor feels comfortable with her own sexual responsiveness (Scale 8). Her high Scale 8 score, which indicates that her desired level of pleasure far exceeds her actual pleasure across many SII items, might on the surface be taken as reflecting a desire to change. While this may be true, we might also reasonably expect Mrs. B to be experiencing a good deal of stress at the present time because of the fact that she appears to find sex unpleasant to the point of aversion. Certainly her sexual self-confidence and self-esteem would warrant careful investigation, and one might suppose that she could require a good deal of support. It would not be out of line to consider that she is depressed to a greater or lesser extent.

In terms of their attitudes toward one another, Scales 5 and 11 indicate that neither partner considers the other ideal. Of the two, Mr. B is the more critical in this respect. This apparent problem is further compounded by poor perceptual accuracy on his part (Scale 4), which unfortunately suggests that Mr. B may actually be overestimating his wife's enjoyment of sexual activity. She, on the other hand, seems well aware of his sexual preferences (Scale 10). This situation is somewhat different from that presented in the case of the As, since here it is only one partner (Mr. B) who seems to be misperceiving things. Since he errs in the direction of overestimating his wife's pleasure, the prospective therapist might tentatively formulate two alternative hypotheses to test during her or his initial contact with the Bs: either Mr. B is ignoring his wife's evident displeasure, or else she is reticent to reveal the depth of her aversion to him.

The Bs' total disagreement score is extremely high, which only adds weight to the hypothesis that their therapist will be confronted by an extremely dysfunctional relationship. Clearly this is *not* the sort of preorgasmia which is likely to respond well to a straightforward shaping and desensitization paradigm.[8]

Again the final piece of data is provided by the Marriage and Sex Defensiveness scales. For Mr. B these scores were 15 and 2, respectively; for Mrs. B they were 15 and 12. Whereas both marriage defensiveness scores are above the mean, they are so by less than one standard deviation. Mrs. B's sexual defensiveness score, however, is nearly two standard deviations above the mean, while Mr. B's score is actually lower than the mean. One might tentatively infer, then, that this couple is fairly straightforward with respect to disclosing general marital conflict but that Mrs. B is actually understating her level of sexual discomfort in responding to our assessment devices.

To summarize, assessment data (again collected prior to therapist-client contact) would lead the prospective therapist to anticipate a difficult case. The presenting complaint of primary inorgasmia, taken by itself, might lead one to proffer a favorable prognosis and to anticipate

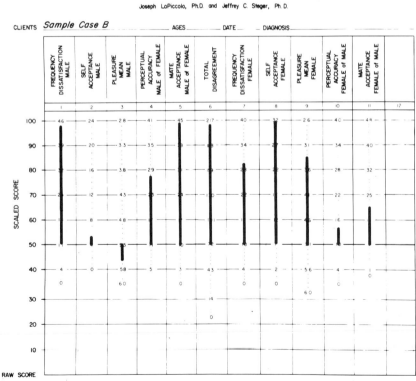

TABLE 5
SEXUAL INTERACTION INVENTORY
Joseph LoPiccolo, Ph.D. and Jeffrey C. Steger, Ph.D.

using a straightforward treatment strategy. In the present case, however, the clinical picture is complicated, and one might well modify both prognosis and treatment strategy. There is strong suggestive evidence to the effect that the female partner of this couple responds to sexual contact with distaste and that she feels abused by her mate. The partners would appear to have divergent goals, he wanting more sexual activity of every kind, she wanting just the opposite. Finally, while one might speculate that Mr. B feels sexually frustrated, his wife suffers additionally from low self-esteem and has yet to reveal to her husband the full extent of her dissatisfaction. While each of these speculations requires confirmation from additional sources of data, most notably the therapist, pretreatment assessment has again provided information which is likely to affect treatment substantively.

SUMMARY

In writing this paper we began with two goals in mind. The first was to describe the kind of clinical assessment of couples that is routinely done at the Stony Brook Sex Therapy Center. Our second goal was to illustrate these procedures through the presentation of sample cases. We are convinced that formal behavioral assessment not only can serve an evaluative research function, but also can materially improve clinical practice. In this latter area of clinical application it is our opinion that behaviorally oriented assessment procedures have a potential that has yet to be realized.

The types of instruments described here, which have been derived largely from a behavioral theoretical perspective, do not require a highly trained professional for administration. On the contrary, they can be administered through the mail and can be easily scored by clerical personnel. The subsequent modest investment of therapist time yields a wealth of significant information. This information bears on the overall quality of the clients' relationship, the nature of their sexual relationship, individual sexual functioning, and potential areas of conflict; it materially affects clinical practice. The therapist possessed of this data may be able to anticipate client resistances and formulate a tentative treatment plan to deal with them. She or he can plan the initial contact so as to investigate "trouble spots" efficiently and with a minimum of random "searching." The end result is a more complete and accurate diagnosis and a treatment plan which has a maximum chance of success.

The amount of useful information that practicing clinicians can gain from standard application of instruments such as those described here can be expected to increase with practice. Yet to be able to extract such hypotheses as typified by the two sample cases presented here requires only a modicum of experience with the tests.

Recent years have seen a proliferation of behaviorally oriented personality assessment devices, some of which are specifically useful for the assessment of sexual behavior in couples. These instruments have potential as effective and efficient aids to those concerned with the treatment of marital and sexual problems. It remains to those who are motivated to pursue this potential.

REFERENCES

1. Rotter JB: Some implications of a social learning theory for the prediction of goal directed behavior from testing procedures. *Psychol Rev 67*:301–316, 1960.
2. LoPiccolo J, Steger JC: The Sexual Interaction Inventory: A new instrument for assessment of sexual dysfunction. *Arch Sex Behav 3*:585–595, 1974.
3. Goldfried MR, Sprafkin JN: *Behavioral Personality Assessment*. Morristown, NJ, General Learning Press, 1974.
4. Locke HJ, Wallace K: Short marital adjustment and prediction tests: Their reliability and prediction. *Marr Fam Living 21*:251–255, 1959.
5. Kimmel D, Van der Veen F: Factors of marital adjustment in Locke's marital adjustment test. *J Marr Fam 29*:57–63, 1974.
6. Locke HJ: *Predicting Adjustment in Marriage: A Comparison of a Divorced and a Happily Married Group*. New York, Holt, 1951.
7. Jemail, JA: Response bias in the assessment of marital and sexual adjustment. Unpublished doctoral dissertation, State University of New York at Stony Brook, 1977.
8. LoPiccolo J, Lobitz WC: The role of masturbation in the treatment of primary orgasmic dysfunction. *Arch Sex Behav 2*:163–171, 1972.

Journal of Sex & Marital Therapy
Vol. 5, No. 3, Fall 1979

The DSFI: A Multidimensional Measure of Sexual Functioning

Leonard R. Derogatis, PhD, and Nick Melisaratos, MHS

ABSTRACT: The present report summarizes work to date on the Derogatis Sexual Functioning Inventory (DSFI), a multidimensional measure of human sexual functioning. We discuss the rationale for the test as well as the selection of the primary domains of measurement. Reliability coefficients for the various subtests are given, and a review section on validation studies is provided, including a factor analysis, predictive validation, and discriminant function analyses. Prototypic clinical profiles are also provided for several of the major types of sexual dysfunction.

In the development of the Derogatis Sexual Functioning Inventory (DSFI) major considerations were initially focused on the feasibility of the enterprise, given the important requirement that the instrument would have to possess clinical relevance and utility. The essential question we addressed was whether we could build a scale that not only measured sexual behavior, but did so in a fashion that would render the product useful to professionals charged with making essential clinical decisions.

Having answered this question in the affirmative, we then moved on to a series of complex technical questions. The first of these decisions concerned the *subject measurement unit:* would we measure males, females, individuals, couples, heterosexuals, homosexuals, or all of these. We decided to utilize the individual as the subjective unit and to develop a normative foundation based upon male and female heterosexuals. In doing so, we did not intend to exclude measurement of other groups with the DSFI, but rather we were responding to the necessity to be specific concerning *whom* it was we were measuring. As it has developed (see the

Dr. Leonard R. Derogatis is Director of the Division of Medical Psychology and the Director of Research of the Sexual Behaviors Consultation Unit of the Johns Hopkins University School of Medicine, and is Associate Professor of Medical Psychology and Associate Professor of Oncology. Nick Melisaratos is a candidate for the degree of Doctor of Science at the Johns Hopkins University School of Hygiene and of Public Health, and Research Associate in the Department of Psychiatry of the Johns Hopkins University School of Medicine. Reprint request should be addressed to Dr. Leonard R. Derogatis, Henry Phipps Psychiatric Clinic, Room 500, The Johns Hopkins Hospital, Baltimore, Maryland, 21205.

0092–623X/79/1500–0244$00.95

Validation section of this paper), the DSFI has proven sensitive with other than male and female sexual dysfunctions, and, theoretically, norms could be developed for any group for whom the items and subtests of the instrument appear relevant.

The next question we addressed concerned the *conceptual measurement continuum:* this issue had to do with the *what* of measurement. Although on initial examination the answer to this question might appear very straightforward, there are in actual fact many different dimensions of sexual activity one could report upon. Capacity for sexual functioning, frequency of sexual behavior, satisfaction with sexual activities, sexual accomplishments, and an enormous number of other distinct but related concepts could all be utilized to create a measurement continuum. We decided upon "current sexual functioning" as the conceptual continuum for the DSFI. We chose this concept because it comes closest to the central question the clinician attempts to answer in the initial evaluation of the patient: What is the current level of sexual functioning of this individual? It has the additional advantage of easily reflecting any positive changes in quality of sexual behavior that may be effected by intervention as well as any inhibiting influences upon sexual functioning from one period to the next. There is also the additional advantage that reports concerning current behavior, fantasy, and feelings are apt to be more accurate than those dependent on long-term memory.

The *measurement modality* was a third important issue that we considered in the development of the DSFI. In the instance of sexual behavior, this comes down to the question of whether to adopt clinician ratings or self-report. The self-report mode of measurement possesses a number of distinct advantages as well as some inherent limitations. Probably the most significant advantage of self-report is that it reflects the phenomena under investigation in terms of the experiencing person himself, i.e., the patient. All other modalities are limited to "apparent" report since they depend upon the skill of the observer in questioning and observing the patient concerning his experiences. Self-report also carries with it cost efficiency, particularly in terms of professional time. Administration, scoring, and initial screening assessments can usually be accomplished by a paramedical or technical assistant, and substantial amounts of clinical data can be delivered to the professional in a format highly amenable to review and assimilation in a brief time span. In addition, the self-report mode lends itself readily to actuarial scoring,[1] and the data may be readily incorporated within clinical decision systems.[2,3]

On the negative side, Wilde[4] reminds us that the use of the self-report mode tacitly assumes the validity of the "inventory premise," that is, that the patient can and will accurately describe the cognitive, affective, and behavioral events of interest to us. We know that this may not always be the case; response biases, such as social desirability,[5] can influence the veridicality of the patient's response. Nonetheless, reports by Rorer[6], Norman,[7] and Fiske[8] make it clear that response biases tend to act rather selectively, with more influence on social traits and when response alternatives are not clearly specified. Considering all of the above reasons, we developed the DSFI in self-report mode.

The final major design question of concern with the DSFI was the dimensionality of the instrument: should we develop a homogeneous unidimensional measure of sexual functioning or a more complex and, of necessity, lengthier multidimensional scale? The unidimensional approach to measurement possesses several characteristics to speak for it: it takes fewer test items to provide a reliable and valid measure of a single construct and thereby can result in a shorter instrument. Unidimensional scales are typically easier to administer and to score, and thereby more cost efficient. If the concept of interest is amenable to continuum measurement without elaboration of the status of other relevant constructs, then a unidimensional model can be the approach of choice.

Unfortunately, the major strength of unidimensional measures in certain situations, i.e., their simplicity and ease of administration, can become a weakness in other contexts. Particularly if the phenomenon under investigation is complex, it is often inadequate and inappropriate to attempt assessment solely through a unidimensional scale. The result is often a fair approximation at best: at worst, it can be a significant distortion of the clinical reality.

In the multidimensional approach to measurement, the construct underlying the conceptual measurement continuum (e.g., current sexual functioning) is operationalized via a linear model that assumes the overall score is the sum of a series of component scores. Each component score has a weight associated with it (in most instances the weight for each component is assumed as 1) and is designed to reflect an important dimension or domain of the global measurement construct.

Although psychometrically and clinically more complex and more time-consuming, multidimensional scales carry with them numerous advantages. First, they provide information on not only the overall status of the individual, but also on various aspects of his functioning, highlighting strengths and weaknesses. They thereby provide a pattern to the individual's behavior as well as a single quantitative summary score. Second, multidimensional models enhance interpretation of test data at multiple levels: overall level of functioning is provided by the global score, while at the next interpretive level primary dimension scores provide a broad-brush profile of the individual's functioning. Should the clinician wish detailed information on issues such as specific experiences, symptoms, or fantasies, the discrete items of the subtests may be reviewed and evaluated.

Finally, multidimensional measurement can provide higher predictive efficiency, particularly in measurement areas where subtests are not highly correlated. Also, these instruments articulate nicely with multidimensional statistical models that can deliver powerful evaluations of nosologic, prognostic, and treatment-outcome questions. Since we believe sexual functioning to be a complex aspect of human behavior, with identifiable and measurable subdomains, and the costs of the multidimensional approach appeared outweighed by the advantages, we adopted a multidimensional model for the DSFI.

SUBSTANTIVE DOMAINS OF THE DSFI

The most demanding effort by far in the development of the DSFI was the selection of the primary substantive domains and the development of a suitable measurement model for each. A combination of clinical experience, broadly based theory, and empirical research all went into the selection of our substantive domains, and even with this effort we were to find our first domain collection inadequate. (In the original 1975 version of the DSFI there were only eight subtests. Body Image and Satisfaction subtests were added to the revised version in 1978, and the number of the Fantasy subtest items was reduced to 20 from 35.)

The DSFI was designed to be an "omnibus" test of sexual functioning, sampling and measuring the major components essential to sexual behavior. By its very nature the test will contain too many subtests to please some and be missing some important aspect of sexual activity according to others. This situation is inevitable in designing such a test, particularly when a time frame of 45-60 minutes is imposed. We believe that the essential components of human sexual functioning are reflected by the DSFI and that its degree of comprehensiveness will ultimately be decided by the collective impact of its empirical validation studies.

The domains selected for inclusion in the DSFI are listed below, and in the section that follows we attempt to provide an appreciation of why each was chosen.

    I. Information
   II. Experience
  III. Drive
  IV. Attitudes
   V. Psychological Symptoms
  VI. Affects
 VII. Gender Role Definition
VIII. Fantasy
  IX. Body Image
   X. Sexual Satisfaction

Information

Although the fundamental drives and mechanisims underlying sexual behavior are under neuroendocrine control[9] and biologically determined,[10] the specific behaviors and activities that comprise the sexual repertoire of mamalian species are predominantly learned behaviors. At the level of humans, accurate information concerning the physiology, anatomy, and psychology of sexual relationship seems essential (at least at its most fundamental levels) for successful and satisfying sexual union.

It is difficult to estimate how many people are inadequately informed regarding sexual functioning, in large measure because there is no consensus regarding what minimum level of sexual information is required to conduct oneself adequately sexually. Culture almost certainly plays a role here; however, we do know that Masters and Johnson[11] cite lack of accurate information as the major cause of sexual dysfunction in their experience. They have since modified their position somewhat,[12] regarding the exclusivity of information lack as the sole cause of dysfunction, but it retains a prominent place in their thinking regarding sexual dysfunction. Derogatis and Meyer[13] have observed statistically significant decrements in the amount of accurate sexual information possessed by sexually dysfunctional men and women; however, they have questioned the clinical significance of this observation due to the small magnitudes of these differences.

In any case, it is certainly logical to assume that the quality of information available regarding sexual behavior correlates to some positive degree with the degree of success one enjoys engaging in it. This may be particularly true in disadvantaged or undereducated groups, and we may find that the weight assigned this component changes as we move through socioeconomic levels. The DSFI measures sexual information through 26 true-false items.

Experience

It is not surprising to anyone that the sexual experience repertoire of any patient presenting with sexual dysfunction is one of the essential elements of the clinical history. Impotence occurring in a shy man of 20 who has never successfully engaged in coitus previously, and has had few opportunities to do so, must be viewed differently than the same complaint emanating from a man of 55 who has had a successful marital relationship for 30 years, with no sexual difficulties at all in a pre- and a number of extramarital relationships.

It is interesting to note that a number of investigators have observed that sexual experiences tend to assume a hierarchical structure.[14-17] if proportional experience is utilized as a criterion. Derogatis, Melisaratos, and Clark[18] confirmed this observation for the judged rank of sexual behaviors as well as a proportional endorsement continuum and further supported Zuckerman,[17] and Bentler[15,16] in their findings of very high correlations (i.e., .95) between male and female hierarchies. Additionally, in an extension of this research, Derogatis, Melisaratos and Clark[19] observed substantial differences in the impact that the experience of various sexual behaviors had on their ranking in the hierarchy, with particular differential effects between males and females.

The level of experience an individual has had sexually correlates positively with reported degrees of success and satisfaction in sexual relationships. It is important data to have in assessing the nature and magnitude of a dysfunction, and it is essential information in evaluating the impact of any intervention. The list of 24 sexual behaviors that comprise the Experience Subtest of the DSFI range from very basic sexual activities to various forms of intercourse and oral-genital behaviors. They provide a reasonable spectrum of experiences across which to conduct a clinical evaluation and their hierarchical relationships have been well studied.

Drive

The concept of sexual or erotic drive is, of course, fundamental to any consideration of sexual functioning. As a construct requiring the development of a measurement model, however, drive presents some unique problems. To begin with, although there are numerous behaviors that are explicitly sexual and therefore appear to be *prima facie* manifestations of erotic drive, we know that sexual behaviors may be motivated by other than sexual needs. Anger, guilt, jealousy, revenge, as well as many other motives, may be the primary underlying forces behind sexual behavior; the cataloging of sexual activities in and of itself does not insure that we are measuring sexual drive.

Conversely, not all libidinal erotic impulses are necessarily translated into explicit sexual behaviors, even if one extends the term behavior to include thoughts and fantasies. Psychodynamic investigations have made it abundantly clear that certain actions, thoughts, feelings, and dreams may serve libidinal purposes but have no explicitly manifest sexual content—these are highly symbolized reflections of erotic drive.

Our solution to this dilemma was to opt to measure explicit sexual behavior, recognizing that our assessment of drive would, of necessity, be imperfect. This choice was made due to the fact that there are an infinity of possible symbolic sexual representations, while only a very finite number of representative sexual activities exists, and they lend themselves nicely to available measurement models.

In operationalizing our measure of drive we adopt an approach somewhat analogous to that taken by Kinsey in his work. Kinsey and his associates[20,21] utilized a composite definition of drive which he termed *total sexual outlet;* this score reflected contributions from autoerotic, heterosexual and homosexual activities. The Drive Subtest of the DSFI is modeled after Kinsey's concept to the extent that it, too, is a summary measure composed of five components. Sexual intercourse, masturbation, kissing and petting, sexual fantasy, and ideal frequency of intercourse all contribute to the overall measure of drive.

Each class of behaviors is measured on a 9-point frequency scale, and these values are summed to produce a total score. Although this measure does miss some of the more subtle manifestations of drive, it is highly correlated with clinical impressions and has revealed high discriminative sensitivity.

Sexual Attitudes

It will come as no surprise that sexual attitudes was selected as one of the domains that is important to our appreciation of quality of sexual functioning. In their "value expressive" function[22] an individual's attitudes concerning sexual activities provide us with insight into his/her sociocultural background. The mores of society as a whole, and the significant subcultural units (e.g., family, peers) in which the individual holds membership, are communicated through attitude postures about sexuality.

We are also aware that attitudes serve a "gating" function in that they may act to screen selective information that is in conflict with the individual's predominant value orientation. Athanasiou[23] refers to this aspect of attitudes as their "ego-defensive" function. This function relates attitudes to affects and thus may provide the clinician with a window on the conflicted aspects of an individual's sexuality. It is most important to have a valid appraisal of a patient's attitudes about sex so that therapeutic communications are not presented in a fashion to produce a direct confrontation with value systems.

In operationalizing a measure of attitudes the psychometrician must narrow the field of focus from "attitudes" to some aspects of attitudes that are less inclusive but retain predictive power regarding sexuality. The constructs that appear best suited for such a role are those of *liberalism* and *conservatism.* These constructs have often been represented as polar opposites, but it appears to be more realistic to depict them as orthogonal dimensions in cartesian coordinate fashion. A patient or individual can then be assigned as a point in two-dimensional space.

There is a good deal of empirical evidence to suggest that these reflections of sexual attitudes possess predictive validity for sexual functioning. Athanasiou and Shaver,[24] as well as other investigators,[25] have consistently shown that persons scoring high on liberalism also show high arousal to sexually explicit material. Individuals showing high conservatism—who currently appear older and less well educated—tend to react with dysphoria and disgust to such explicit depictions and have been characterized by Mosher and Greenberg[26] as experiencing higher levels of guilt about sexual behavior. The score of the Attitude Subtest on the DSFI is actually a difference score (liberalism-conservatism) with 15-item scales defining each of the two major constructs. The subtest is scored in a fashion to weight higher liberalism scores positively for adequate sexual functioning.

Psychological Symptoms

There should be little need to communicate the notion that a comprehensive clinical evaluation requires the assessment of the degree and nature of psychopathology present. Although it is sometimes difficult to determine the antecedent versus resultant status of psychological disorders seen in the sexually dysfunctional patient, the requirement to obtain a reliable appraisal of any psychopathology present is no less necessary.

There are some difficulties inherent in the self-report modality regarding psychological symptoms; however, the majority of patients will accurately report their experiences of psychological distress. In particular, patients presenting for a sexual dysfunction are not usually seriously (e.g., psychotically) disturbed, and they tend to be highly motivated to obtain relief from their sexual difficulties. Although there are exceptions, the majority of patients will provide accurate reports of their emotional problems.

In recent years one of the major issues in the literature surrounding sexual dysfunctions has been the question of the degree of psychological disorder and disintegrity implied by the sexual disorder. Classical psychoanalytic writers (e.g., Fenichel,[27] Ferenczi[28]) typically portrayed sexual dysfunctions as serious disturbances, "the tip of the iceberg," reflecting deep-rooted neurotic and characterologic problems. Other investigators, although they may differ as to precisely how disturbed they believe sexual dysfunctions to be, also characterize them as revealing inordinate levels of psychological disturbances.[13,29–32]

In opposition to this idea Masters and Johnson[11] have described the majority of their patients with sexual dysfunctions as being free of any formal psychiatric disorders. In holding this view they concur with other investigators[33–36] who have also failed to observe a significant relationship between sexual dysfunction and neurotic disorders.

Since this question is of significant consequence, and to some degree the lack of consonance on this issue is due to inadequate measurement of psychopathology in some studies, we decided to employ a complete psychometric test to measure psychopathology on the DSFI. The Symptoms Subtest of the DSFI is comprised of the Brief Symptom Inventory

(BSI), which is the brief (53-item) form of the SCL-90-R.[38,39] The BSI takes approximately 10 to 12 minutes to complete and is itself a multidimensional scale that may be scored and displayed in terms of nine primary symptom dimensions* and three global indices of distress. The General Severity Index (GSI), one of the global measures from the BSI, is the symptom component which contributes to the overall DSFI score. Much of the work discussed in the subsequent section on validation indicates that our choice of employing a more complete measure of psychopathology was a wise one.

Affects

One of the most striking clinical characteristics of patients who present with sexual dysfunctions is the profound level of dysphoric affect they manifest. Both males and females with sexual disorders display a wide range of negative emotions that are readily discernible clinically. Disordered sexuality typically results in marked unhappiness for those afflicted, often with a sense of being trapped and unable to escape this very perplexing and self-deprecating disability.

From another vantage point many experts in human sexuality have commented on the etiologic significance of negative affects. Lazarus,[40] discussing the causal bases of impotence, has written, "They all boil down to one single basic cause—negative emotions." He cites guilt in particular as being an affect state instilled by society regarding sexual behavior, and Derogatis[32] has characterized guilt as a "conditioned emotional response (CER) prescribed by society as the correct response to stimuli of a sexual nature." Similarly, Cooper[34] and Lidberg[41] have thoughtfully discussed the etiologic role of anxiety in sexual disorders, while Fisher and Osofsky,[42] Mellan,[43] Lewis,[44] and Gutheil[45] speak to the causal impact of anger and resentment in sexual dysfunctions. Depression has been consistently related to sexual dysfunction etiologically, through a mechanism that Klein[46] describes as a "deranged pleasure center." He further portrays the fundamental cause as "a sharp, unreactive, pervasive impairment of the capacity to experience pleasure or respond affectively to the anticipation of pleasure."

Because dysphoric affect is such a pervasive concomitant of sexual disorders and because of its etiologic significance, we decided that affects on the DSFI should also be measured by a proven psychometric instrument. Our choice was to measure affects via the Affects Balance Scale (ABS)[47] a brief adjective checklist which has proven sensitive to clinically

---

*The nine primary symptom dimensions of the BSI are somatization (SOM), obsessive-compulsive (O-C), interpersonal sensitivity (INT), depression (DEP), anxiety (ANX), hostility (HOS), phobic anxiety (PHOB), paranoid ideation (PAR), and psychoticism (PSY).

initiated mood differences in a number of distinct contexts[13,48,49] The ABS is an unobtrusive scale comprised of 40 adjectives which are scored in terms of four positive and four negative affect dimensions.* Positive and negative totals are subsequently generated, and the difference between them—the Affect Balance Index—is the score that contributes to the DSFI. As is the case with the Brief Symptom Inventory, the ABS may be scored and displayed in a multidimensional format.

Gender Role Definition

For the majority of the present century masculinity and femininity were considered polar opposites on a single conceptual continuum. More recent research, with both animals[50] and humans[51] suggests that a more accurate conceptualization involves viewing masculinity and femininity as distinct orthogonal dimensions on which every organism assumes a relative position early in life. Therefore, we are not either masculine or feminine, but both masculine *and* feminine. The translation of the relative balance between these two patterns of behavior becomes established as an individual's *gender identity,* and, as Money and Erhardt[52] state, "gender role is the public expression of gender identity".

Money[53] writes, "The differentiation of a core gender identity probably follows the same principle as the differentiation of the gonads and the internal reproductive organs. In other words, two systems are present to begin with, only one of which becomes fully functional." The other system does not regress to trace status, however, as it does in the case of reproductive systems, but rather through the mechanism of "complementation" becomes an alternate gender schema utilized in the prediction and response to the other sex gender-coded behavior patterns.

It is through the related processes of identification and complementation that gender role definition plays a significant part in sexual functioning. The polarized gender role definition, be it masculine or feminine, not only prescribes a rigid delineation of the role model anticipated for self, but through the mechanism of complementation also carries with it a very specific pattern of behaviors for the sexual partner. Deviations from or dissatisfaction with prescribed role behaviors on the part of the partner seriously jeopardize the well-being of individuals with polarized gender role definitions. For this reason these persons are substantially more prone to difficulties with sexual dysfunction (see, e.g., Derogatis, Meyer and Dupkin[54]).

In developing a measure of gender role definition we adopted an

---

*The positive primary affect dimensions of the ABS are joy (JOY), contentment (CON), vigor (VIG), and affection (AFF): the primary negative affect dimensions are anxiety (ANX), depression (DEP), guilt (GLT), and hostility (HOS).

approach similar to that of Bem.[51] Our gender role measure is a difference score, resulting from the algebraic difference between femininity and masculinity scores. Each of these dimensions is viewed as orthogonal and is, in turn, reflected by 15 gender-stereotyped adjectives that have been previously assessed as to their degree of societal gender stereotype. Gender role definition has a significant influence upon sexual functioning, even though it may be subtle, and it is essential that the effects of this influence be measured and appraised.

Sexual Fantasy

Along with sexual behavior, one of the pivotal reflections of erotic urges and drives are sexual fantasies. May[55] has commented, "Fantasy is the language of the total self, communicating, offering itself, trying on for size . . . if one cannot do this *he* will not be present in the situation, sexual or other, whether his body is there or not. Fantasy assimilates reality and then pushes reality to a new depth."

From the clinician's viewpoint fantasy is important because it provides a window on the sexual wishes and drives of the patient. He can learn which of these the individual is comfortable in acting out behaviorally and which are restricted only to the realm of reverie. From a patient's fantasies we can learn not only of his conflicts and frustrations, but also his most sought after desires. The "rehearsal" function of fantasy provides the opportunity to choreograph sexual behavior in daydreams and can communicate to the clinician the presence of disruptive themes of anxiety or guilt. Contemporary cognitive behavior therapies are effective, in part, due to reprogramming the internal dialog of the individual toward a more productive rendition of the "scene."

In addition to its rehearsal function, fantasy can also serve to achieve "vicarious fulfillment." Situations which are essentially unobtainable in actuality may be engaged in the realm of fantasy. As a variation of this aspect of fantasy, Hariton and Singer[56] have pointed out that fantasy may be utilized as a "creative enrichment" of real-life sexual situations which are less than optimal. In either case, evaluation of the patient's sexual fantasy life can add much to our clinical assessment and should be accomplished in a systematic fashion.

Our own Fantasy Subtest consists of 20 major sexual themes that have been culled from material on normal sexual functioning as well as clinical variations on sexual activities. At present, only a very rudimentary score, which consists of simply counting the number of fantasy themes endorsed by the patient, is used on the DSFI. We soon hope to have large enough samples to develop a set of weights for the fantasy themes that maximally separate disordered from normal sexual functioning. In the interim we are evaluating fantasies configurally as well as using the summed score.

Body Image

A positive self-concept is an important element in a healthy adjustment to society and the environment, reflecting objective self-assessment and reality testing unencumbered by need-induced distortions. In addition, a positive evaluation of self carries with it a measure of autonomy and a clear sense of environmental mastery. Thus, self-esteem is promoted by a self-image that includes a capacity for loving and being loved, proven abilities and accomplishments, and a potential for dealing effectively with the challenges presented by life.

Sexual relationship is one of the very significant life challenges faced by human beings and is also often one of the more profound vehicles for the expression of love and affection. In addition, the sense of being a complete "man" or "woman" is also based to a large degree on the ability to conduct successful sexual relations. In our experience one of the most pervasive obstacles to achieving a relaxed and conducive posture in sexual relationship is physical self-deprecation or negative body image.

Even before Schilder's[57] pioneering work on body image, it was abundantly clear that one's impression of one's own body can have a profound effect on an individual's self-concept. As Schilder notes, it is not only a single direct self-evaluation of physical attractiveness that one must deal with, but also the "reflected perceptions" of others around us who are the final arbiters of perceived physical beauty.

We know that in extreme cases of physical disfigurement, including congenital defect,[58] surgical interventions such as colostomy[59,60] and pelvic exenteration,[61] and trauma such as amputation,[62] or spinal cord injury,[63] there are significant negative alterations in body image that coincide with reductions in self-esteem and difficulty readjusting. What is not so apparent is that many people without any ostensible physical decrement or trauma, nonetheless, possess extremely negative and deprecating images of their physical bodies.

This is possible, in part, because body image is formed rather early in development and depends heavily upon other reflected evaluations of one's beauty. Hartman[64] in his classical ego studies has pointed out that positive investment in one's physical body is a function of childhood pleasure or displeasure derived from peer evaluations of physical attractiveness. The curious puzzle of confronting a beautiful adult patient who is ruminatively concerned about some self-perceived physical deficiency may be partially explained by the fact that at an earlier time (i.e., in childhood) her body was a source of embarrassment and humiliation to her rather than of joy and enhancement. Subsequent alterations in physical attractiveness cannot erase the initial insult to self-esteem; they may only cover it over and in doing so take on a transient quality which constantly reminds the individual of "from whence she came."

Our Body Image Subtest on the DSFI consists of 15 items—10 common items plus 5 unique items each for males and females. The individual is required to rate himself/herself on 10 general body attributes, which are the same for both sexes, and an additional 5 gender-specific items that are focused more specifically on satisfaction with genital attributes. This simple subscale has proved most sensitive in discriminating dysfunctional status, and we anticipate it will show a broader profile of validity in future work.

Satisfaction

On the surface, the issue of sexual satisfaction appears quite straightforward: either an individual *is* or *is not* satisfied with his/her sexual relationships. More detailed evaluation tells us, however, that sexual satisfaction has a number of distinct but related facets. *Frequency* of sex and the degree of *variation* in sexual activities are two major themes regarding sexual satisfaction that are repeatedly put forward. Often an individual desires sex more frequently than his partner, or wishes to be more adventurous than his partner cares to be. In many instances these two aspects of satisfaction are observed to be correlated, with low-drive individuals also being less invested in sexual novelty.

Communication between sexual partners, or rather the lack thereof, is a frequent theme of sexual dissatisfaction, particularly concerning some aspect of coitus. Often a partner will complain that *foreplay* was not arousing or did not last long enough or that intercourse itself was too brief. Failure to achieve *orgasm* is, of course, a very frequent complaint, particularly among women; however, men too may experience orgasm as unpleasant or be incapable of achieving it (e.g., in retarded ejaculation). The *resolution* phase of sex is often found to be less than satisfactory for one or both partners, even though we frequently spend little clinical time exploring this aspect of sexuality. Some patients complain of a lack of feeling fulfilled, while others do not experience the sense of relaxation they seek.

In still other instances the problems with sexual satisfaction exists at a broader level: the individual may feel that his/her partner is no longer sexually gratifying as a person, that it is not the details of sexual performance that are dissatisfying but the interpersonal relationship with the partner itself. Obviously, it is important to know this since the nature of the intervention recommended would depend upon it greatly.

Recognizing these distinctions, we framed them into 10 items on the DSFI to provide a glimpse of the individual's degree of satisfaction sexually and the aspects of sexuality that give rise to it. Obviously, sexual satisfaction is a complex domain; however, we hope to gain an insight into it with the Sexual Satisfaction Subtest of the DSFI.

RELIABILITY

The reliability of an instrument essentially speaks to the problem of consistency of measurement. In the self-report mode there are two forms of reliability that concern us primarily: *internal consistency* and *test-retest*. The former addresses the question of consistency with regard to *homogeneity* of items, that is, to what degree do the items which comprise a certain dimension of the test fall together or show commonality in their operational definition of the construct being measured. Internal consistency reliability reflects the average correlation between items.

Test-retest reliability reflects consistency in a different fashion; here consistency or precision in measurement is defined in terms of *stability*. Test-retest reliability focuses on the degree of correlation between test scores at two different points in time. It is essential for an instrument to have good test-retest reliability over the time spectrum that it is utilized to make predictions.

If we examine the subtest and component coefficients provided in Table 1, we can see that reliability for the various subtests of the DSFI is quite good. Both internal consistency and test-retest coefficients tend to be very high and well within the acceptable range. There are some differences in the particular components for which we generated either internal consistency or test-retest coefficients which needs clarification.

Since Attitude, Affect, and Gender Role subtest raw scores are each essentially difference scores, determined by subtracting the score on one homogeneous dimension (e.g., masculinity) from another homogeneous orthogonal dimension (i.e., femininity), it did not appear logical to investigate the internal consistency of the actual subtest score. Rather, what is of interest is the homogeneity of the components. A similar logic was utilized concerning the Symptoms subtest where we have nine components instead of two.

Overall, internal consistency reliability was very good for the DSFI, with various subtest measures such as Experience and Fantasy revealing very high coefficients. The major component scores (e.g., liberalism, conservatism; positive affect, negative affect, masculinity, femininity) also showed very high internal consistency for their part. On those subtests where coefficients were a bit lower (e.g., Drive and Body Image) we would not expect from our appreciation of the construct and the design of the subtest to obtain very high coefficients. Thus, we know that items on frequency of intercourse, masturbation, and sexual fantasy on the

TABLE 1
Internal Consistency and Test-Retest Reliability Coefficients for the Subtests of the DSFI

Subtest	Number of Items	Internal Consistency[a] (N=325)	Test-Retest[b] (N=60)
I Information	26	.56	.61
II Experience	24	.97	.92
III Drive	5	.60	.77
IV Attitude	30	---	.96
a. Liberalism	15	.81	.92
b. Conservatism	15	.86	.72
V Symptoms[a]	53	---	.90
VI Affect		---	.81
a. Positive Total	20	.93	.75
b. Negative Total	20	.94	.42
VII Gender Role		---	.84
a. Masculinity	15	.84	.60
b. Femininity	15	.76	.58
VIII Fantasy	20	.82	.93
IX Body Image	15	.58	---
X Satisfaction	10	.71	---

[a]Internal Consistency Coefficients for the 9 primary symptom dimensions of the BSI are as follows: Som= .80, OC= .83, Int= .74, Dep= .85, Anx= .81, Hos= .78, Phob= .77, Par= .77, Psy= .69

[b]Test-Retest coefficients are based on a 14-day retest interval

Drive Subtest to some degree tap "unique" aspects of sexual functioning as well as some that are common to the construct "sexual drive." Our Body Image Subtest has two distinct components—one focused on general physical appearance while the other measures satisfaction with genital anatomy more or less. It is quite possible that these two subsets of items may reflect two distinct aspects of body image to some degree. The coefficient for the Information Subtest does fall below acceptable levels somewhat, indicating that this subtest may require reanalysis.

Turning to our test-retest coefficients, we again must come to the general conclusion that in terms of stability of measurement the DSFI performs admirably. Experience, attitude, symptoms, and fantasy coefficients are all over .90, while those for affect and gender role are above .80. The retest coefficient for drive is also relatively high, at .77. The affect component coefficients are reduced somewhat; however, this is precisely what one would expect from fluctuating measures of mood.

Our information coefficient was also lower than desired on the stability measure, and this result coupled with our internal consistency measure suggests that we may need modifications on this subtest. It is possible that certain items are too difficult for our population resulting in high levels of guessing on those items and subsequent reductions in homogeneity and stability scores.

On the whole, however, the reliability evaluations for the DSFI are quite good. While we will continue to investigate and attempt to improve our precision of measurement, we believe present levels are more than adequate to achieve meaningful clinical prediction with the test.

VALIDATION

The validation of a psychological test is a programmatic exercise that requires multiple studies and years to accomplish. In one sense, the validation of a test is perpetual in that each new predictive context the test is used in requires separate validation. In practice, we tend to fall back on the generalization of previous validation situations to the one we are currently working in, assuming that it contains no unique factor or influence that would diminish the sensitivity of our instrument. Even at that, validation still requires much effort and many studies before one feels comfortable talking about a valid test.

The material appearing in this section is from a continuing series of studies with the DSFI attempting to demonstrate its predictive validity in a number of clinical situations and, ultimately, to demonstrate its construct validity.[65,66] Some of this work has been reported previously.[18,19,32,48,54,67,68] Other work is currently in press.[13,69,70] The remainder is data which are principally reported for the first time here with our "new" sample ($N = 380$). A detailed demography of the sample—male and female sexual dysfunctions and male and female non-patient normals—appears in Table 2. It also should be noted that the revised version of the DSFI (i.e., 10-subtest version) was not in the field in time to be used with all the individuals in this sample, and so, some data deal only with the original (8-subtest) version of the scale.

Internal Structure of the DSFI

In developing a multidimensional measure of a complex construct like "current sexual functioning," its various components are usually represented as orthogonal or uncorrelated. This is usually because of ease of presentation and, in part, because such a depiction represents an idealized measurement model. In the clinical worl such components or domains are almost always correlated to some degree, often quite markedly.

TABLE 2
Demographic Characteristics of a Sample of 380 Sexual Dysfunctions
and Non-Patient Normals

	MALE		FEMALE	
	Normals (N=76)	Dysfunctions (N=91)	Normals (N=154)	Dysfunctions (N=59)
Age	$\bar{x}$= 31.40 σ= 9.07	$\bar{x}$= 41.21 σ= 12.37	$\bar{x}$= 32.33 σ= 8.96	$\bar{x}$= 31.52 σ= 9.54
Race	%	%	%	%
White	88.1	91.0	76.7	96.4
Black	10.2	9.0	21.8	3.6
Religion				
Catholic	33.9	31.0	21.7	34.5
Protestant	32.2	29.9	39.5	38.2
Jew	6.8	12.6	24.8	9.1
Other	8.5	6.9	4.7	7.3
No Affiliation	18.6	19.5	9.3	10.9
Marital Status				
Single	33.9	23.1	33.3	8.9
Divorced	1.8	11.0	6.8	5.4
Separated	1.8	9.9	3.8	5.4
Widowed	0.0	1.1	1.5	0.0
Married	62.5	54.9	54.5	80.4
Social Class				
I	12.3	11.2	16.0	14.5
II	42.1	21.3	49.6	25.5
III	38.6	37.1	27.5	25.5
IV	7.0	22.5	4.6	21.8
V	0.0	7.9	2.3	12.7

Thus, even though symptoms and affects are two totally independent conceptualizations, when we view them in term so individuals, we will most certainly observe them to be highly correlated. This being the case, it is a worthwhile and an important exercise to investigate the empirical dimensions of the instrument and determine how well they conform to the hypothesized rational constructs underlying them.

To accomplish this, we conducted a principle components analysis on the pooled data from our sample of 380 subjects. To facilitate interpretation, the original solution was rotated to a normalized varimax criterion. Male and female sexual dysfunctions as well as nonpatient normals comprised the sample. In selecting variables we did not limit ourselves to the 10 primary domain scores: rather we utilized component scores in some instances (e.g., masculinity-femininity), and in the case of drive, used the seven basic drive item scores. Our reasoning here was that we would learn much more about the actual internal structure of the instrument and avoid forcing arbitrary interpretations. Twenty-one measures were utilized in this fashion, and results of the analysis appear in Table 3.

Seven interpretable factors were derived from the analysis which accounted for 52 percent of the variance in the matrix. The largest of those, accounting for almost 20 percent of the variance, was labeled "psychological distress." The interpretation of this dimension was relatively uncomplicated by virtue of the fact that the two psychological symptom measures (i.e., GSI and PSDI) and the negative affects measure loaded heavily on it, while positive affects revealed a substantial negative loading on this factor. Factor II had only two variables loading on it strongly, body image and the GSSI. It has become increasingly obvious that body-image evaluation is an integral aspect of sexual functioning, a fact which gains further support from its high correlation with self-rated global sexual satisfaction (i.e., the GSSI). Due to its singular correlation with the body measure this factor has been labeled "body image."

Factor III is represented primarily by drive items pertaining to frequency of intercourse and kissing and petting behaviors and, to a lesser extent, by degree of sexual experience, and by ideal frequency of sexual intercourse. The GSSI also shows a moderate loading on this dimension. This collection of variables reflects the extent of involvement and investment in heterosexual relationships and activities, as well as level of satisfaction with sexual functioning. For this reason we have labeled the dimension "heterosexual drive."

Factor IV is an interesting dimension in that it reflects items that have to do with self-stimulating erotic behaviors. Masturbation, frequency of sexual fantasy, and variety of sexual fantasies are the sole items that correlate with this dimension. It appears to be reflecting a distinct aspect of sexual behavior other than those requiring a partner's participation, and we have labeled this dimension "autoeroticism."

Factor V has been labeled "gender role" because both masculinity and femininity scores load on this factor, with differences in the strengths of the loadings possibly resulting from the somewhat disproportionate composition of the sample. In addition, the positive affects component also shows a strong correlation with this factor. Positive correlations for both gender dimensions and positive affect bring to mind Bem's[71] observation that low scores on both gender components tend to correlate with low self-esteem. It is possible that this factor reflects general self-concept, but at the moment it is too soon to tell.

Factor VI has only a single variable comprising it and that is "satisfaction." In a most interesting fashion, satisfaction as measured by our 10 specific items does not correlate highly with other dimensions but appears to reflect a somewhat unique dimension of sexuality.

Factor VII is comprised of two items from the Drive Subtest—"age at first interest in sex" and "age at first intercourse." Neither of these items

TABLE 3

Orthogonal Varimax Loadings for 7 Factors Generated from a Principal Components Analysis of 21 Measures on the DSFI [a]

No.	Variable	I Psychological Distress	II Body Image	III Heterosexual Drive	IV Autoeroticism	V Gender Role	VI General Satisfaction	VII Sexual Precociousness
1.	Information	–	–	–	–	–	–	–
2.	Experience	–	–	.36	–	–	–	–
3.	Drive- Intercourse	–	–	.76	–	–	–	–
4.	Drive- Masterbation	–	–	–	.52	–	–	–
5.	Drive- Kissing & Petting	–	–	.78	–	–	–	–
6.	Drive- Fantasy	–	–	–	.54	–	–	–
7.	Drive- Ideal Frequency	–	–	.35	–	–	–	–
8.	Drive- First Interest	–	–	–	–	–	–	.37
9.	Drive- First Intercourse	–	–	–	–	–	–	.66
10.	Liberalism	–	–	–	–	–	–	–
11.	Conservatism	–	–	–	–	–	–	–
12.	Symptoms-GSI	.86	–	–	–	–	–	–
13.	Symptoms-PSDI	.72	–	–	–	–	–	–
14.	Affects- Positive	-.49	–	–	–	.62	–	–
15.	Affects- Negative	.74	–	–	–	–	–	–
16.	Femininity	–	–	–	–	.75	–	–
17.	Masculinity	–	–	–	–	.36	–	–
18.	Body Image	–	-.92	–	–	–	–	–
19.	Fantasy	–	–	–	.58	–	–	–
20.	Satisfaction	–	–	–	–	–	.72	–
21.	GSSI	-.36	-.74	.39	–	–	–	–
	a^2	4.00	2.25	1.37	1.10	0.92	0.75	0.47
	% Variance	19	11	7	5	4	4	2

[a] Only loadings above .35 are represented

is normally scored on the subtest, but they are evaluated configurally and used for research purposes. Their tendency to reflect a small unique dimension of their own without high correlation with other measures suggests that they might be reflections of another unique dimension of human sexuality and possibly serve as core items of a separate dimension. We have labeled this factor "sexual precociousness."

Clinical Characteristics of the DSFI

As mentioned previously, the validation of a psychological test instrument ultimately depends upon its ability to separate one clinical group of interest from another. Some groups are very distinct from each other (e.g., transsexuals vs. normals), and therefore easy to separate, while others are much more alike (e.g., impotent males vs. premature ejaculators) and demand greater discriminative power from the test instrument. We have chosen in this section of the report to demonstrate the predictive validity of the DSFI by demonstrating its ability to separate one clinical group from another. In most instances the comparisons will be between nonpatient normals and sexual dysfunctions; however, in a few cases other comparisons will be alluded to in an effort to clarify or sharpen a particular point.

In our recently completed contrast of a sample of 150 sexual dysfunctions with a comparison group of 230 nonpatient normals, the demography of the two samples was compared. With the exception of our male patients being significantly older and our female patients more frequently married, the demography of the two samples was generally comparable.

Statistical evaluations of the differences in DSFI and subtest scores were conducted for males and females separately and are summarized in Tables 4 and 5. Graphic DSFI profiles for the two comparisons are presented in Figures 1 and 2.

Taking the males first (Table 4, Figure 1), we see a very marked difference in the Sexual Functioning Index scores for the two groups with dysfunctional males manifesting a mean score of approximately 434 compared to the normal mean of 513. This global score places our male dysfunctionals almost 2σ below the normative mean, at approximately the fifth centile of sexual functioning. The comparison group of nonpatient normals is $.5\sigma$ above the mean in their DSFI overall scores.

Female dysfunctions (Table 5, Figure 2) also reveal a significant reduction in their DSFI scores, although their mean value of 446 is not quite as reduced as their male counterparts. This value places them approximately 1.5σ below the normative mean for females.

Reviewing the components of the profile, we observe significant differences between our normal and dysfunctional males on 9 of the 10

TABLE 4

Means, Standard Deviations and t-Values for Male Sexual Dysfunctions vs. Male Normals
on the Subtests and Globals of the DSFI

Subtest	Non-Patient Normals (N=76)		Sexual Dysfunctions (N=91)		t	p
	x̄	σ	x̄	σ		
I Information	21.20	2.14	19.42	3.21	4.13	.001
II Experience	20.77	4.04	17.93	4.79	4.07	.001
III Drive	18.64	5.96	14.89	6.05	4.02	.001
IV Attitude	27.21	13.45	23.87	14.50	1.53	n.s.
V Symptoms	.44	.36	.61	.46	-2.67	.01
VI Affect	1.72	.79	.84	1.00	6.14	.001
VII Gender Role	-8.33	8.43	-4.86	9.90	-2.41	.02
VIII Fantasy	7.36	4.55	5.75	3.78	2.49	.01
IX Body Image[a]	11.72	5.44	20.56	6.05	-4.40	.001
X Satisfaction[a]	7.82	1.60	5.34	2.11	3.63	.001
DSFI Score	513.16	44.26	433.91	34.98	7.57	.001
GSSI	5.19	1.53	2.47	1.56	11.01	.001

[a]Sample sizes were smaller for this subtest since it was introduced
after the trials were initiated.

subtests. Only on the attitudes subscale do we fail to see a significant difference between the groups. Females, on the other hand, do not reveal as many significant distinctions between the normal and dysfunctional groups. Significant differences were observed on information, symptoms, affects, body image, and satisfaction but were not in evidence on the other dimensions.

Looking at differences on the Information Subtest, we notice marked statistical differences for both sexes, an observation we have consistently made in other research.[3,48,70] Masters and Johnson[12,13] have repeatedly pointed to information decrement as a pivotal etiologic factor in sexual disorders, and although we did not see heavy loadings for this subtest in our internal structure analysis (see the "internal structure" discussion in the validation section), it does emerge as a significant contributor in our clinical discriminant studies (see the following "discriminative capacity" discussion in this section).

Experience was also a significant discriminator between male dysfunctions and normals although it did not distinguish among females. Sexual experience decrement has been observed previously with dysfunctional males; with male and female "invested partners,"[69] however, this subtest has not shown reductions for female dysfunctions.[13]

In Table 6 we have listed the specific items from the Experience Sub-test that revealed significant differences between the two male groups. Eleven different activities showed significant reductions in proportional endorsements between the two male groups. All 11 behaviors were also observed to discriminate dysfunctional males in a previous study, along with 3 additional behaviors that were not significant here.[13] As previously reported, these males tend to show decrements in more "advanced" sexual experiences, e.g., various forms of intercourse and oral-genital behaviors. This finding suggests that dysfunctional males may not be adventurous or creative sexual partners; however, it is difficult to know whether that is cause or effect relative to the sexual problem.

On the Drive Subtest we again observe a situation where the measure discriminates among males but not among females. Dysfunctional women have drive levels approximately equivalent to normals, while men show a significant reduction. In order to obtain a better appreciation of this difference, we examined the actual items of the subtest. Table 7 displays the endorsement frequencies of males for the two items that were significantly different—intercourse and ideal frequency of intercourse. On the

TABLE 5

Means, Standard Deviations and t-Values for Female Sexual Dysfunctions vs. Female Normals on the Sub-Tests and Globals of the DSFI

Subtest	Non-Patient Normals (N=154)		Sexual Dysfunctions (N=59)		t	p
	$\bar{x}$	σ	$\bar{x}$	σ		
I Information	21.31	2.72	20.22	2.86	2.58	.01
II Experience	20.05	4.54	19.19	4.66	1.24	n.s.
III Drive	16.54	6.68	15.73	7.76	.76	n.s.
IV Attitude	20.63	14.45	18.91	15.63	.76	n.s.
V Symptoms	.46	.42	.65	.52	-2.66	.01
VI Affect	1.55	.81	.72	1.18	5.88	.001
VII Gender Role	-.57	7.88	.53	8.69	-.88	n.s.
VIII Fantasy	4.51	3.39	4.97	3.67	-.87	n.s.
IX Body Image[a]	14.66	4.44	20.11	5.21	-2.68	.01
X Satisfaction[a]	8.89	1.05	4.21	2.20	6.02	.001
DSFI Score	503.00	29.27	446.53	42.13	5.98	.001
GSSI	4.81	2.20	2.34	1.48	7.97	.001

[a]Sample sizes were smaller for this subtest since it was introduced after the trials were initiated.

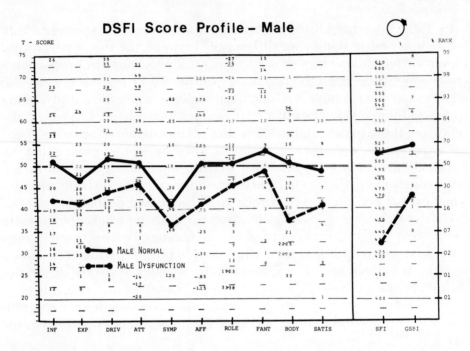

FIGURE 1: DSFI Profiles of 91 Sexually Dysfunctional Males and 76 Male Nonpatient Normals.

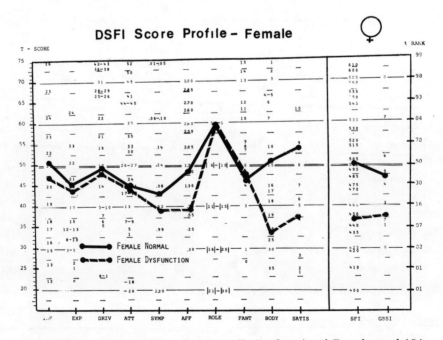

FIGURE 2: DSFI Profiles of 59 Sexually Dysfunctional Females and 154 Female Nonpatient Normals.

TABLE 6
Proportional Endorsements of Items in the Experience Subtest
For Male Normals and Dysfunctions

Item	% Normals Endorsing	% Dysfunctions Endorsing	x^2	p
1. Male lying prone on female (clothed)	94.7	72.5	12.48	.001
3. Erotic Embrace	96.0	82.4	6.20	.01
4. Intercourse- vaginal entry from rear	78.7	58.2	6.91	.01
7. Oral stimulation of partner's genitals	88.0	72.5	5.13	.02
8. Intercourse- Side by Side	90.7	62.6	15.90	.001
10. Intercourse- Sitting position	73.3	50.5	8.03	.004
16. Intercourse- Female Superior Position	90.7	73.6	6.78	.01
17. Mutual petting of genitals to orgasm	82.7	58.2	10.40	.001
19. Mutual undressing of each other	92.0	75.8	6.56	.01
20. Deep Kissing	98.7	86.8	6.44	.01
21. Intercourse- Male Superior Position	96.0	83.5	5.40	.02

TABLE 7
Frequencies of Endorsement of the Two Items From the Drive Subtest That
Discriminates Male Sexual Dysfunctions From Male Normals

Code	Frequency	Sexual Intercourse		Ideal Frequency of Intercourse	
		% Norm	% Dysf	% Norm	% Dysf
0	Not at all	5.3	25.3	3.9	13.2
1	Less than once per month	3.9	22.0	1.3	5.5
2	1-2 times per month	19.7	15.4	6.6	4.4
3	Once a week	15.8	12.1	10.5	7.7
4	2-3 times per week	39.2	22.0	21.1	34.1
5	4-6 times per week	18.4	0.0	32.9	15.4
6	Once a day	1.3	0.0	13.2	7.7
7	2-3 times per day	1.3	2.2	7.9	6.6
8	4 or more per day	0.0	1.1	2.6	5.5
x^2		42.12		16.74	
p		.001		.03	

former we see over 47 percent of the dysfunctional group reporting intercourse "less than once per month" while a comparable percentage among normals is 9 percent. On "ideal frequency" 19 percent of dysfunctionals endorsed "less than once per month", while only 5 percent of normals did so. From this data we can see that it is the motivation specifically for intercourse that is reduced among dysfunctional males and not drive in general.

The Symptoms Subtest reveals significant elevations for both dysfunctional men and women when compared to normals. Dysfunctional males reveal a mean GSI score about 1.3σ above (literally on the profile, "below") the normative mean, and even though our sample of male normals also is somewhat elevated, the dysfunctions reveal significantly more distress than the normals. A similar picture emerges for the females. Dysfunctional females have a mean score 1.1σ above the normative mean, and even though our female comparison sample also shows somewhat of an elevation, it is significantly below that of the dysfunctions.

Our research group has long been interested in the issue of psychopathology among dysfunctional patients and has repeatedly observed clinical levels of psychological symptoms in this group.[13,32,68] In one report encompassing 359 dysfunctional patients[68] we established prototype symptom profiles for the three major nosological categories of impotence, premature ejaculation, and anorgasmia.

In general, all three groups showed elevated profiles between 1 and 1.5σ. Impotent males manifested highest distress levels, with peaks on depression and anxiety, and secondary elevations on somatization and psychoticism. The latter essentially reflects alienation in this sample, with little of the scores arising from severe or first-rank symptoms. Premature ejaculators revealed a less dramatic profile, which was, nonetheless, significantly raised. Their highest scores were on anxiety and hostility measures. Anorgasmic females fell slightly below the impotent males in terms of overall levels of distress. They revealed peaks primarily on depression and interpersonal sensitivity, the latter a syndrome of negative self-concept, self-depracating thoughts, and inferiority feelings, akin to the old concept of "inferiority complex." Anorgasmic females also manifest clear symptoms of alienation.

Although we have not plotted a multidimensional profile for our dysfunctional patients in the present sample, perusal of their BSI scores indicates their profiles would be little different from those just discussed. Although we cannot say whether these symptoms arise from or contribute to the dysfunction, we can confidently say that there are substantial levels of psychological distress among patients with sexual dysfunctions.

This distress also extends to the partners of individuals with sexual dysfunction, at least to males forced to play this role.[67]

The last statement is amply borne out by our comparisons of the groups on affects. Both male and female dysfunctions have mean affects scores that are 1σ below the normative mean. Clinically, the profound levels of unhappiness experienced by these individuals is most striking, and our present evaluations amply bear this out. Previous research with male transsexuals,[48] female transsexuals,[70] and sexual dysfunctions[13] has revealed consistent reductions in positive affect when comparisons are made to control groups, with concomitant elevations in negative affect dimensions. Anxiety, depression, guilt, and hostility are all observed at significantly higher levels in individuals with sexual disorders, suggesting a pervasive quality to their anhedonia. These mood disturbances should not be taken lightly; rather they should be thoroughly investigated and dealt with in the therapeutic interaction.

Research on gender role definition and gender identity has expanded rapidly in the last 5 to 10 years, given particular impetus by the work of Money and Ehrhardt[52] in psychoendocrinology and Bem[51] psychometrically. Our work in this area has shown the concept of gender role definition to have high predictive value in many aspects of human sexuality. Figure 3 is taken from some of our work with male and female transsexuals[48,70] and clearly shows hyperpolarization of each of the gender dysphoric samples on the Gender Role Subtest score of the DSFI.

Present findings indicate that the gender role score significantly discriminates male dysfunctions from male normals, but is not successful in separating the female groups. Male dysfunctions revealed less masculine (i.e., less negative) role definition on the DSFI than normals although this decrement was not marked (approximately $.5\sigma$). Female dysfunctions reveal scores that are essentially androgenous and balanced as a group and differ little from our comparison group scores. A previous study indicated no significant difference between dysfunctions and controls for either sex on the gender role score; however, significant reductions in both component scores were observed.[13] Our interpretation of this finding is in line with Bem's[71] hypothesis of reduced self-esteem for individuals with low scores on *both* masculinity and femininity.

Results with the Fantasy Subtest essentially repeat and amplify our previous findings.[13] In that study we observed a disordinal interaction between sex and dysfunctional status, with male dysfunctions showing reductions in sexual fantasy compared to normals, while dysfunctional females actually showed higher levels of sexual daydreaming. These effects were weak and statistically marginal, however. In the present com-

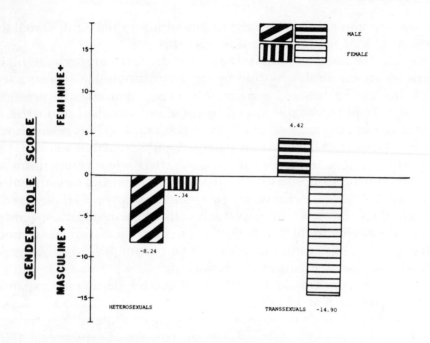

FIGURE 3: Mean Gender Role Scores for 31 Male and 20 Female Transsexuals Compared to Normative Samples of Male and Female Normals.

parison dysfunctional males revealed significantly lower levels of sexual fantasy than normals, and female dysfunctions again revealed greater levels; however, this latter effect did not reach statistical significance.

In our previous evaluation of this finding we observed that the particular fantasy themes proportionally absent among dysfunctional males were those dealing with manifestly carnal scenarios. "Forcing a sexual partner to submit," "degrading a sexual partner," "having intercourse in unusual positions" were typical of the kinds of fantasies less likely to be observed among males with sexual dysfunction. One explanatory hypothesis might be that the dysfunction had impaired these males' confidence in their masculinity and sexual assertiveness to such a degree that they were unable, even in reverie, to assume an active carnal posture.

Evaluation of the nature of female dysfunctions' fantasies also proved interesting. The scenarios where they showed proportional increases over normal females tended to be more liberal and unfettered by sexual convention. Our provisional explanatory hypothesis regarding this result is similar to Hariton and Singer's[56] "creative enrichment" hypothesis, whereby the unfulfilled female seeks a cognitive enhancement of her dissatisfying actual experience through mental embellishments. It is not clear, however, whether this behavior is dependent on a cognitive "style," which is evident in many life activities as these authors suggest, or is a mechanism specific to sexual activities.

The Body Image Subtest is one of the "new" scales recently added to the revised DSFI. This domain of behavior was included in the test because clinical assessments and therapeutic interactions repeatedly suggested that body image relates in a very fundamental way to sexual functioning. The results of our comparisons bear this hypothesis out dramatically. Particularly among male dysfunctions, but also among female disorders, we see profound decrements in body image scores. Both male and female dysfunctional patients reveal mean body image values approximately 1.5σ below the normative mean; this places them, on the average, in the bottom 10 percent of the population.

A graphic representation of the difference between dysfunctions and normals on this measure is given in Figure 4. As is obvious from these smoothed curves of the respective distributions for males, body image is an axis of discrimination for individuals with sexual disorders.

A more detailed evaluation of items that showed differences between patients and normals indicated that dissatisfaction with general body features as well as displeasure with genital attributes contributed to the differences. Our evaluation of the internal structure of the test (see the first section of the validation discussion) indicated that body image represented a salient dimension of the DSFI, and our subsequent analysis has pointed to its being a powerful discriminator as well.

Satisfaction was the other new domain added to the revised DSFI for the reason outlined earlier in this report. We could not escape the conclusion that sexual satisfaction is a complex multidetermined aspect of sexual functioning that would continue to remain elusive unless some means of objectifying it were introduced. Although it does not come as a surprise, we were pleased to observe very significant differences between sexual dysfunctions and normals on the Satisfaction Subtest. Differences were highly significant for both males and females, with dysfunctions' mean scores falling from 1.00 to 1.25σ below the normative mean.

In order to provide greater insight into the specific aspects of satisfaction that were reported as deficient by our dysfunctional samples, we analyzed responses on an item-by-item basis. Those items that revealed significant differences are recorded in Tables 8 and 9.

The predominant aspect of sexual satisfaction that provides difficulty for male dysfunctions is "worry over performance," which is reported by almost 89 percent of the male patients. To a lesser degree, "orgasm" itself provides a problem, and quality of "communication with partner" is also

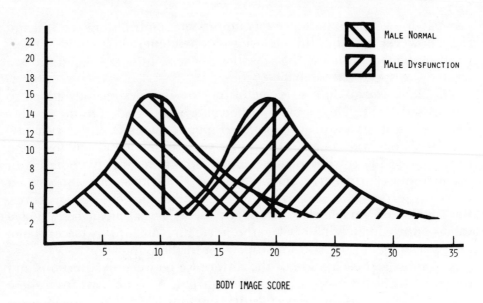

FIGURE 4: Body Image Score Distributions from the DSFI for 98 Male Sexual Dysfunctions Contrasted with 69 Male Normals.

the basis for dissatisfaction. Among female dysfunctions, dissatisfaction is more broadly based, but the overwhelming sources of dissatisfaction are quality of "orgasm" and lack of a sense of "fulfillment". As may be seen from Table 9, 7 of the 10 items show significant differences between female dysfunctions and normals on this subtest. We have known for some time (Meyer, 1975) that a significant difference in the bases of male and female sexual dysfunctions lies in the fact that the former are primarily performance oriented while the latter are disorders of satisfaction.

TABLE 8
Proportional Endorsements of the Satisfaction Subtest
Items for Male Normals and Dysfunctions

Satisfaction Item	% Normals In Agreement	% Dysfunctionals In Agreement	x^2	p
7.I have satisfying orgasm	91.7	56.8	3.58	.05
9.I worry about sexual performance	25.0	88.6	17.1	.001
10.Good Communication with my partner about sex	91.7	56.8	3.58	.05

TABLE 9

Proportional Endorsements of the Satisfaction Subtest Items for
Female Normals and Dysfunctions

Satisfaction Item	% Normals In Agreement	% Dysfunctions In Agreement	x^2	p
1. Satisfied with Sexual Partner	100.0	36.8	7.53	.005
4. After sex I feel relaxed, fulfilled	81.8	18.2	16.91	.001
6. I am not very interested in sex	0.0	47.2	4.29	.04
7. I have satisfying orgasm	77.8	15.8	7.70	.005
8. Foreplay is very arousing	100.0	47.4	5.25	.02
9. I worry about my sexual performance	11.1	63.2	4.72	.03
10. Good communication with my partner about sex	100.0	52.6	4.30	.04

Our present results could not be much stronger in supporting this notion.

Discriminative Capacity of the DSFI

In the final analysis, an assessment instrument is only as good as the "incremental validity"[73] it brings to the clinical decision situation. That is to say, it must contribute some unique predictive information that is not available from other sources; otherwise it is redundant and its costs in time and energy cannot be justified.

In an attempt to assess the discriminative sensitivity of the DSFI, we subjected profiles of normals and sexual dysfunctions to discriminative function analyses—separately for males and females. Unfortunately, at the time the study was conducted, the "new" samples on the revised DSFI were not available, and as a result these analyses were done with the original (eight-subtest) DSFI samples reported elsewhere.[13] The analyses were conducted on the SPSS system[74] using a forward stepwise algorithm; they are summarized in Tables 10 and 11.

Essentially what the analyses reveal is that the DSFI is capable of making discriminant assignment at levels substantially above chance. The classification matrices reveal 77 percent correct assignment among males and 75 percent correct assignment among females. Since chance alone would result in 50 percent correct assignment, we see an approximate 25 percent increase in predictive efficiency.

Examination of the discriminant coefficients reveals that with both males and females information, symptoms, affects, and fantasy are the

TABLE 10
Discriminant Analysis of Male Sexual Dysfunctions vs. Male Normals via the
8 Subtests of the DSFI

Discriminant Function Classification	Classification by Diagnosis			Standardized Discriminant Coefficients	
	Normal	Dysfunctional			
Normal	43 (75.4%)	14 (24.6%)	57	Information	.256
				Drive	.361
Dysfunctional	10 (21.3%)	37 (78.7%)	47	Symptoms	.318
	53	51	104	Affects	.960
				Fantasy	.171

Total Correct Assignment = 77%

subtest scores that contribute significantly to the discrimination. In addition, drive scores also contribute significantly in the case of males. Negative affects contribute conspicuously to the discrimination between the two groups, supplemented by drive scores among the males and symptom scores among the females.

In all probability we would anticipate "shrinkage" in our discriminant capacity when the equations are utilized in subsequent cross-validation

TABLE 11
Discriminant Analysis of Female Sexual Dysfunctions vs. Female Normals via the
8 Subtests of the DSFI

Discriminant Function Classification	Classification by Diagnosis			Standardized Discriminant Coefficients	
	Normal	Dysfunctional			
Normal	111 (77.6%)	32 (22.4%)	143	Information	.299
				Symptoms	.709
Dysfunctional	14 (35%)	26 (65%)	40	Affects	1.281
	125	58	183	Fantasy	-.165

Total Correct Assignment = 75%

samples; it must be remembered, however, that this result was obtained on an early version of the instrument, missing two important subtests. It is our expectancy that the distinct contribution of body image and satisfaction to our discriminant ability would more than compensate for any shrinkage that would result.

DSFI CLINICAL PROFILES

In spite of the most sophisticated psychometric analyses, and veritable mountains of data addressing the issue of validation in numerous contexts, for the clinician much of this data retains a technical, academic quality. The clinician requires an assessment mechanism that delivers sufficient amounts of relevant information in a short period of time, preferably without having to read through pages of clinical reports.

The answer to this need, at least in terms of psychological tests, comes in the form of the *clinical psychometric profile*—a picture or graph that summarizes the patient's status on the relevant variables of measurement and plots them out in relation to each other. Essentially, the raw score distribution on each of the measurement dimensions are converted over to a comparable standardized score distribution (e.g., T-scores with $\bar{X} = 50$; $\sigma = 10$), and then plotted consecutively to create a pattern. From this the clinician may glean how profound the disturbance is, the strengths and weaknesses of the patient, and his characteristic psychosexual attributes.

Although a few profiles are far from sufficient to enable the professional to gain a complete clinical understanding of the use of the DSFI, they do enable one to establish a feel for the test and the nature of the information it communicates.

A Case of Premature Ejaculation

Mr. T is a 28-year-old white male referred to our clinic by a psychiatrist for evaluation and treatment of premature ejaculation. He was one of four children in a Catholic family, himself a college graduate and working in sales. He has known and dated his wife for approximately 8 years, the last 4 of which they have been married. Mr. T has been premature in all sexual relationships with women, and with his wife since their first attempts together. They realized there was a problem early in their relationship but felt somehow they would work it out. More recently he has become somewhat obsessed with his sexual dysfunction, and the couple's relationship is beginning to show signs of strain. There are no formal psychiatric or medical diagnoses of either member of the couple, although she has become increasingly dysphoric with weight loss recently. Attempts at sexual union have dwindled to less than once a month from a previous frequency of once per week.

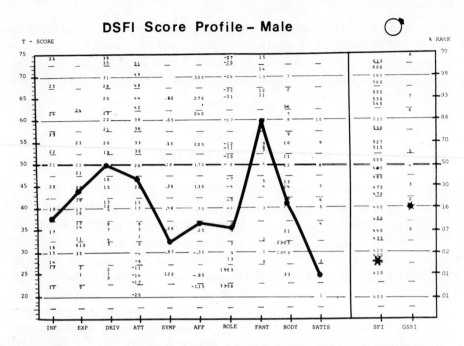

FIGURE 5: DSFI Profile of a 28-Year-Old White Male Suffering from Premature Ejaculation.

In evaluating Mr. T's profile we can see that his overall DSFI score of 418 is more than 2σ below the mean, placing him in the bottom 1 to 2 percent of the population. His own estimate of his level of current sexual functioning (i.e., the GSSI) is given as "highly inadequate." This is somewhat atypical for premature ejaculators in that they usually do not have such negative overall assessments.

Evaluating his profile, we see substantial decrements on information, experience, symptoms, affects, gender role, body image, and satisfaction. Drive levels remain unimpaired, which in this case, are attested to by the high levels of sexual fantasy. His attitude posture, although somewhat conservative, is well within functional limits. The low information levels and reduction in sexual experiences suggest the patient has had limited sexual exposure. Although he speaks vaguely of other encounters, it is possible that his wife has been his only sexual partner. Symptom levels suggest mild to moderate psychological distress, with affect clearly dysphoric. Gender role scores are in a range formally classified as "androgenous"; however, low scores on both masculinity and femininity dimensions may indicate a problem with self-esteem.[71] Although not profound, we see evidence of body image decrement which is diffuse and consistent with generally lowered self-esteem. The patient's satisfaction score is extremely low, and strongly suggests that this couple may be dealing with a broader problem than merely Mr. T's premature ejaculation. A detailed evaluation of the Brief Symptom Inventory (i.e., the Symptom Subtest) shows clinical elevations on interpersonal sensitivity, depression, anxiety, and alienation, which may reflect a fundamentally insecure individual who is caught in a serious conflict about his adequacy as both an individual and a sexual partner.

A Case of Impotence

Mr. W is a 50-year-old white male college graduate who has been referred by a urologist to the clinic for psychological evaluation aroudn the presenting problem of impotence. He and his wife have been married for 19 years and report "excellent" sexual relations until 5 years ago. At that time Mr. W began to experience episodic attacks of impotence that became progressively worse. Shifts in sexual habits, increased variety in sexual practices (i.e., the introduction of oral-genital activities), and other forms of experimentation helped temporarily; however, the impotence was progressive and in recent years has been complete (at least with Mrs. W). Mr. W was evaluated via penile tumescene recording in a sleep laboratory and found to have unimpaired nocturnal erectile periods. Mrs. W also reports that her husband has early morning erections, and on several occasions when it was impossible for them to have coitus, he was observed by her to have an erection. A thorough evaluation revealed Mr. W to be suffering from secondary impotence of psychogenic origins, with an absence of any psychiatric or medical diagnosis.

An assessment of Mr. W's results on the DSFI indicates that his score of 400 places him 3σ below the mean. His self-assessment (GSSI) of his sexual functioning is "poor." Mr. W's profile reveals significant decre-

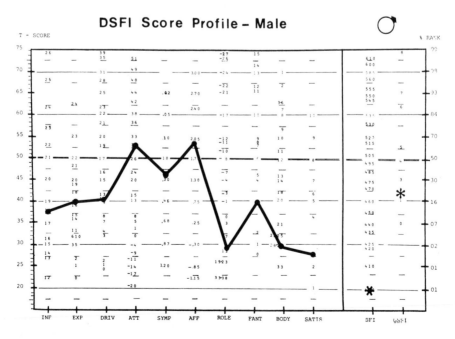

FIGURE 6: DSFI Profile of a 50-Year-Old White Male Suffering from Impotence.

ments on information, experience, drive, gender role, fantasy, body image, and satisfaction. Reductions in levels of both drive and fantasy suggest reduced libido in this patient, probably related to his repeated failure to achieve potency. Interestingly, Mr. W shows low levels of sexual information for a man of his educational background and a certain amount of constriction in the variety of his sexual experiences. We may be dealing here with a man with very limited sexual experience outside that obtained in his marital relationship: Mr. W's gender role score is well into the feminine spectrum and approximately 2σ away from what is considered optimal for male sexual functioning. Body image and satisfaction scores are also more than 2σ below the mean. The relatively positive status of this patient on both the Symptoms and Affects subtests is rather unusual for cases of impotence and suggests that he may not actually be distressed about his dysfunction, indicating the possibility of strong secondary gain.

A Case of Anorgasmia

Mrs. D is a 31-year-old white female who presented to the clinic with the complaint of secondary anorgasmia, referred by her gynecologist. The patient has been married for 10 years and has two children. The patient is a high school graduate and has a position in sales. She claims that for the past several years she and her husband have become increasingly alienated from each other and have not had sex for the past 8 months. Recently, she has been involved with men in a number of casual affairs, which she claims she enjoyed sexually but which did not result in orgasm and have lowered her self-esteem. Mrs. D is extremely conflicted about remaining with her husband but maintains that she is doing it for the children. The patient is extremely articulate and physically very attractive. She indicates experiencing orgasm only a few times in her life, always through manual manipulation. Throughout the interview the patient was affectively quite dysphoric and represented herself somewhat theatrically. She was diagnosed as a secondary anorgasmia with concomitant psychiatric diagnoses of reactive depression occurring in a hysterical personality.

Mrs. D's DSFI score places her current level of sexual functioning at about 1.8σ below the norm. Consistent with her characterologic diagnosis her own assessment of her level of sexual functioning (GSSI) was at the lowest possible level—"could not be worse." Mrs. D's profile shows quite a few areas of strength as well as some problem areas. She has a high level of accurate information about sex and has had a wide range of sexual experiences (often seen in anorgasmias). Her attitude is conducive to good sexual functioning as is her gender role definition. She has an active sexual fantasy life (also seen frequently in anorgasmias), and other measures of drive appear unimpaired. On the negative side, she reveals a very depreciated body image in spite of her physical beauty. This decrement is found in relation to both her general physical appearance and the appearance of her genitals. Symptomatically her BSI reveals that she has a profile consistent with a clinical reactive depression with a deep sense of alienation. The latter is reflected in her very negative affect balance.

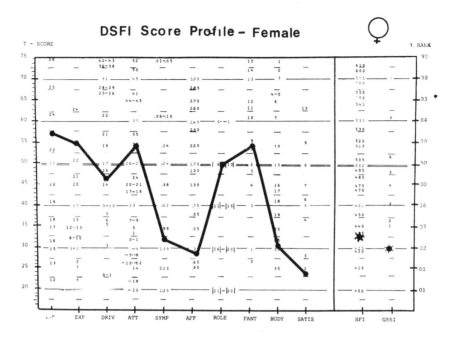

FIGURE 7: DSFI Profile of a 31-Year-Old White Female Diagnosed as Reactive Depression in a Hysterical Personality Suffering from Anorgasmia.

These profiles provide only the smallest sample of the kind of information the DSFI can deliver to the clinical decision enterprise. A great deal more information can also be gleaned from component and discrete item scores which we did not have space to discuss here. It is our hope that ultimately we will be able to develop a detailed clinical interpretive system for the DSFI and make the clinical utilization of the instrument even more productive.

REFERENCES

1. Meehl PE, Dahlstrom WG: Objective configural rules for discriminating psychotic from neurotic MMPI profiles. *J Consult Psychol 24*:375-387, 1960.
2. Fowler RD: Automation and the computer. In JN Butcher (Ed), *MMPI: Research Developments and Clinical Applications.* New York, McGraw-Hill, 1969.
3. Glueck BC, Stroebel CF: The computer and the clinical decision process. *Am J Psychiatry 125*(7) Suppl: 2-7, 1969.
4. Wilde GJS: Trait description and measurement by personality questionnaires. In RB Cattell (Ed), *Handbook of Modern Personality Theory.* Chicago, Aldine, 1972.
5. Edwards AL: *The Social Desirability Variable in Personality Assessment and Research.* New York, Holt, 1957.
6. Rorer LG: The great response-style myth. *Psychol Bull 63*:129-156, 1965.
7. Norman WT: On estimating psychological relationships: Social desirability and self-report. *Psychol Bull 67*:273-293, 1967.
8. Fiske DW: *Measuring the Concepts of Personality.* Chicago, Aldine, 1971.
9. Beach FA (Ed): *Human Sexuality in Four Perspectives.* Baltimore, Johns Hopkins University Press, 1977.
10. Whalen RE: Brain mechanisms controlling sexual behavior. In FA Beach (Ed), *Human Sexuality in Four Perspectives.* Baltimore, Johns Hopkins University Press, 1977.

11. Masters WH, Johnson VE: *Human Sexual Inadequacy.* Boston, Little, Brown, 1970.
12. Masters WH, Johnson VE: Current status of the research programs. In J Zubin, J Money (Eds), *Contemporary Sexual Behavior: Critical Issues in the 1970's.* Baltimore, The Johns Hopkins University Press, 1973.
13. Derogatis LR, Meyer JK: A psychological profile of the sexual dysfunctions. *Arch Sex Behav 8*:201-223, 1979.
14. Podel L, Perkins JC: A Guttman scale for sexual experience—A methodological note. *J Abnorm Soc Psychol 54*:420-422, 1957.
15. Bentler PM: Heterosexual behavioral assessment. I. Males. *Behav Res Ther 6*:21-25, 1968.
16. Bentler PM: Heterosexual behavioral assessment. II. Females. *Behav Res Ther 6*:27-30, 1968.
17. Zuckerman M: Scales for sexual experience for males and females. *J Consult Clin Psychol 41*:27-29, 1973.
18. Derogatis LR, Melisaratos N, Clark MM: Scaling of sexual experiences by direct magnitude estimation. Paper read at the 46th Annual Meeting of the Eastern Psychological Association, New York, April 1975.
19. Derogatis LR, Melisaratos N, Clark MM: Gender and sexual experience as determinants in a sexual behavior hierarchy. *J Sex Marital Ther 2*:85-105, 1976.
20. Kinsey AC, Pomeroy WB, Martin CE: *Sexual Behavior in the Human Male,* Philadelphia, Saunders, 1948.
21. Kinsey AC, Pomeroy WB, Martin CE, Gebhard PH: *Sexual Behavior in the Human Female.* Philadelphia, Saunders, 1953.
22. Katz D: The functional approach to the study of attitudes. *Pub Opin Q 24*: 163-204, 1960.
23. Athanasiou R: A review of public attitudes on sexual issues. In J Zubin, J Money (Eds), *Contemporary Sexual Behavior: Critical Issues in the 1970's.* Baltimore, Johns Hopkins University Press, 1973.
24. Athanasiou R, Shaver P: Correlates of heterosexuals' reactions to pornography, *J Sex Res 7*:298-311, 1971.
25. Wallace C, Wehmer G, Podany E: Contemporary community standards of visual erotica. In *Technical Report* of Committee on Pornography, Vol 9. Washington, DC, U.S. Government Printing Office, 1974.
26. Mosher DL, Greenberg I: Females affective responses to reading erotic literature. *J Consult Clin Psychol 33*:472-477, 1969.
27. Fenichel O: *Psychoanalytic Theory of the Neuroses.* London, Routledge & Kegan, 1946.
28. Ferenczi S: *Sex in Psychoanalysis.* New York, Basic Books, 1950.
29. Lidberg L: Social and psychiatric aspects of impotence and premature ejaculation. *Arch Sex Behav 2*:(2), 1972.
30. O'Conner J, Stern L: Developmental factors in functional sexual disorders. *NY State J Med 72*:1838-1843, 1972.
31. Meyer JK, Schmidt CW, Jr, Lucas MJ, Smith E: Short-term treatment of sexual disabilities: Interim report. *Am J Psychiatry 132*:172-176, 1975.
32. Derogatis LR: Psychological assessment of the sexual disabilities. In JK Meyer (Ed), *Clinical Management of Sexual Disorders.* Baltimore, Williams & Wilkins, 1976.
33. Cooper AJ: Neurosis and disorders of sexual potency in the male. *J Psychosom Res 12*:141-144, 1968.
34. Cooper AJ: Factors in male sexual inadequacy: A review. *J Nerv Ment Dis 149*:337-359, 1969.
35. Maurice W, Guze S: Sexual dysfunction and associated psychiatric disorders. *Compr Psychiatry 11*:539-543, 1970.
36. Faulk M: "Frigidity": A critical review. *Arch Sex Behav 2*:257-266, 1973.
37. Derogatis LR: *The Brief Symptom Inventory.* Baltimore, Clinical Psychometrics, 1975.
38. Derogatis LR: *The SCL-90-R Manual I: Scoring Administration and Procedures for the SCL-90-R* Baltimore, Clinical Psychometrics, 1977.
39. Derogatis LR, Rickels K, Rock AF: The SCL-90 and the MMPI. A step in the validation of a new self-report scale. *Br J Psychiatry 128*:280-289, 1976.
40. Lazarus AA: Psychological causes of impotence. *Arch Sex Behav 2*:39-42, 1972.
41. Lidberg L: Social and psychiatric aspects of impotence and premature ejaculation. *Arch Sex Behav 2*:135-146, 1972.
42. Fisher S, Osofsky H: Sexual responsiveness in women: Psychological correlates. *Arch Gen Psychiatry 17*:214-226, 1967.
43. Mellan J: Interpersonal relationships of female patients with sexual disorders as assessed by Leary's test. *Arch Sex Behav 1*:263-267, 1971.
44. Lewis JM: Impotence as a reflection of marital conflict. *Med Aspects Hum Sex 3*:73-78, 1969.
45. Gutheil EA: Sexual dysfunctions in men. In S Arieti (Ed), *American Handbook of Psychiatry,* Vol 1. New York, Basic Books, 1959.

46. Klein DF: Endogenomorphic depression. Paper presented at International Symposium on Depression, Erbach, Germany, September 1973.
47. Derogatis LR: *The Affect Balance Scale.* Baltimore, Clinical Psychometrics, 1975.
48. Derogatis, LR, Meyer JK, Vazquez F: A psychological profile of the transsexual: I. The male. *J Nerv Ment Dis 166*:234–254, 1978.
49. Derogatis LR, Abeloff MD, Melisaratos N: Psychological coping mechanisms and length of survival in metastatic breast cancer. *JAMA* (in press).
50. Whalen RE: Sexual differentiation: Models, methods, and mechanisms. In RC Friedman, RM Richart, RL VandeWiele (Eds). *Sex Differences in Behavior.* New York, Wiley, 1974.
51. Bem SL: The measurement of psychological androgeny. *J Consult Clin Psychol 42*:155–162, 1974.
52. Money J, Ehrhardt A: *Man and Woman, Boy and Girl.* Baltimore, Johns Hopkins University Press, 1972, p. 4.
53. Money J: Human hermaphroditism. In FA Beach (Ed), *Human Sexuality in Four Perspectives,* Baltimore, Johns Hopkins University Press, 1977, p. 65.
54. Derogatis LR, Meyer JK, Dupkin CN: Discrimination of organic versus psychogenic impotence with the DSFI. *Sex Marital Ther 2*: 229–239, 1976.
55. May R: *Love and Will.* New York, Norton, 1969, p. 281.
56. Hariton EB, Singer JL: Womens' fantasies during sexual intercourse. *J Consult Clinical Psychol 42*:313–322, 1974.
57. Schilder P: *The Image and Appearance of the Human Body.* New York, International University Press, 1950.
58. Easson WM: Psychopathological environmental reaction to congenital defect. *J Nerv Mental Dis 142*:453–459, 1967.
59. Dlin BA, Perlman A, Ringold E: Psychosexual response to ileostomy and colostomy. *Am J Psychiatry 126*:374–381, 1969.
60. Orbach CE, Tallent N: Modification of perceived body and of body concepts. *Arch Gen Psychiatry 12*:126–135, 1965.
61. Lamont JA, DePetrillo AD, Sargeant EJ: Psychosexual rehabilitation and exenterative surgery. *Gynecol Oncol 6*:236–242, 1978.
62. Reinstein L, Ashley J, Miller KH: Sexual adjustment after lower extremity amputation. *Arch Phys Med Rehab 59*:501–504, 1978.
63. Fitting MD, Salisbury S, Davies NH, Mayclin DK: Self-concept and sexuality of spinal cord injured women. *Arch Sex Behav 7*(2):143–156, 1978.
64. Hartmann H: Comments on the psychoanalytic theory of the ego. *Psychoanal Study Child 5*:74–96, 1950.
65. Guion RM: Validates and values in psychological measurement. *Am Psycholog 29*: 287–296, 1974.
66. Messick S: The standard problem: meaning and values in measurement and evaluation. *Am Psycholog 30*:955–966, 1975.
67. Derogatis LR, Meyer JK, Gallant BW: Distinctions between male and female invested partners in sexual disorders. *Am J Psychiatry 134*:385–390, 1977.
68. Derogatis LR, Meyer JK: Psychological symptom profiles of sexual dysfunctions. Paper read at the 4th Annual Meeting of the Eastern Association of Sex Therapists, New York, 1978.
69. Derogatis LR, Meyer JK: The invested partner in sexual disorders: A profile. *Am J Psychiatry* (in press).
70. Derogatis LR, Meyer JK, Boland P: A psychological profile of the transsexual: II. The female (submitted for publication).
71. Bem SL: On the utility of alternative procedures for assessing psychological androgeny. *J Consult Clin Psychol 45*:196–205, 1977.
72. Meyer JK: Individual psychotherapy of sexual disabilities. In AM Freedman, HI Kaplan, BJ Sadock (Eds), *Comprehensive Textbook of Psychiatry,* 2nd ed. Baltimore, Williams & Wilkins, 1975.
73. Sechrest L: "Incremental validity". A recommendation. *Educ Psycholog Measure 23*:153–158, 1963.
74. Nie NH, Hull CH, Jenkins JG, et al: *Statistical Package for the Social Sciences.* New York, McGraw, 1975.

Journal of Sex & Marital Therapy
Vol. 5, No. 3, Fall 1979

The Sex Knowledge and Attitude Test (SKAT)

William R. Miller, PhD, and Harold I. Lief, MD

ABSTRACT: The Sex Knowledge and Attitude Test (SKAT) was designed to measure knowledge, attitudes and degree of experience in a variety of sexual behaviors, and to be used as a teaching and research instrument. The SKAT has been administered to over 35,000 students, approximately two-thirds of whom have been medical students. SKAT has served two major objectives: to measure changes in knowledge and attitudes after a course or program in human sexuality and to demonstrate the deficiencies of medical and nursing education in preparing health professionals to aid patients with sexual problems. Additional types of research using the SKAT are suggested.

DEVELOPMENT OF THE SKAT

The Sex Knowledge and Attitude Test (SKAT) was originally designed in 1967 by Harold I. Lief, MD, and David Reed, PhD, at the Center for the Study of Sex Education in Medicine,[1] Marriage Council of Philadelphia, and the University of Pennsylvania. It was developed as a means of gathering information about sexual attitudes, knowledge, degree of experience in a variety of sexual behaviors, as well as a means of obtaining a diversity of biographical information. It was hoped that the SKAT would be of value as a teaching aid in courses dealing with human sexuality, as a research instrument for the social sciences, and as a self-study aid. Since its publication in 1972, the SKAT has been administered to over 35,000 undergraduates, graduate, and medical students. The test has been used in many countries and has been translated into several languages.

In developing the SKAT, a pool of questionnaire items was drawn from a survey of relevant literature, clinical experience, and socially controversial, sex-related topic areas. This item-pool gave the test its essential

Dr. Miller is Director of Research and Assistant Professor of Psychology in Psychiatry, Marriage Council of Philadelphia, Department of Psychiatry, University of Pennsylvania. Dr. Lief is Director and Professor of Psychiatry, Marriage Council of Philadelphia, Department of Psychiatry, University of Pennsylvania. Reprint requests should be directed to Dr. William R. Miller at the Marriage Council of Philadelphia, 4025 Chestnut Street, Philadelphia, Pennsylvania 19104.

0092-623X/79/1500-0282$00.95

character, in the sense of content areas to be covered. The format of the SKAT items was influenced by three objectives: (1) items would be in either multiple-choice or true-false formats that could be easily scored; (2) there would be measurement of a number of variables through groups of items; i.e., scales; and (3) the items would be potentially usable throughout the entire range of post-high school, higher education.

The current form of the SKAT represents an abridgment and refinement of the original item-pool. The scorable sections of the SKAT, i.e., the attitude and knowledge sections, are the result of administration of preliminary versions of the test to large samples of students, factor analyses, and individual item analyses for internal consistency and item-total score correlations.

The SKAT yields five scores—four attitude and one knowledge score. The Attitude section of the SKAT consists of 35 five-alternative, Likert-type items, and responses to these items result in scores on four attitude scales: Heterosexual Relations (HR), Sexual Myths (SM), Abortion (A), and Autoeroticism or Masturbation (M). The Knowledge section is composed of 71 true-false items, and it yields a single score which reflects the respondent's knowledge of biological, psychobiological, psychological, and social aspects of human sexuality. The biographical information and sexual experience sections of the SKAT are not scored.

ATTITUDE AND KNOWLEDGE SCALES

Attitude Scales

Scores on the four Attitude Scales and on the Knowledge Scale can be obtained either as raw scores or as standardized scores. The standardized scores are *T*-scores with a mean of 50 and a standard deviation of 10 with freshman through senior medical students in the United States as the reference population. Thus, scores between 40 and 60 are within 1 standard deviation from the mean of the score for American medical students. Changes in an individual's or group's attitudes or knowledge over time can be assessed by examining either the raw scores or the standardized scores, although the *T*-scores do offer the advantage of comparison to a standard, reference population.

Factor analyses of both the preliminary and current forms of the SKAT identified four factors underlying the attitude section. Internal consistency reliability (coefficient-alpha) estimates for these scales range from .68 to .86, indicating moderately good to good internal consistency of the SKAT attitude scales. The scales contain seven to nine items each. Three of the items in the attitude section are nonscored "filler" items.

Heterosexual Relations Scale (HR). The HR Scale deals with an indi-

vidual's general attitude toward pre- and extramarital heterosexual behavior. Individuals with high HR scores (above 60) regard premarital
sexual relations as acceptable, or even desirable for both men and
women. These individuals view extramarital relations as potentially bene-
fitting, rather than harming, the marital relationships of those involved.
Low HR scores (below 40) indicate conservative attitudes in this area.

Sexual Myths Scale (SM).   The SM Scale is concerned with the individual's acceptance (low SM scores) or rejection (high SM scores) of commonly
held sexual misconceptions. Included in this scale are items representing
misconceptions about sex education, homosexuality, oral-genital sex, and
determinants of sex drive and sexual responsiveness.

Abortion Scale (A).   The A Scale refers to an individual's general social,
medical, and legal feelings toward abortion. Higher A scores indicate
more liberal attitudes toward and acceptance of abortion.

Masturbation Scale (M).   The M Scale deals with general attitudes toward the permissibility of masturbatory activities. Individuals with high
M scores view autoerotic stimulation as healthy or acceptable, whereas
low M scores indicate that the individuals see masturbation as an un-
healthy practice.

Knowledge Scale

As mentioned above, the knowledge section of the SKAT yields a single
score, reflecting the individual's knowledge of biological, psychobiological, psychological, and social aspects of human sexuality. Since the SKAT
was designed not only as a research tool and self-study aid, but also as a
classroom teaching aid, some of the items in the knowledge section were
included only for their classroom discussion value and not as items to be
included in the total score. Thus, the knowledge section contains 71
true-false items: 50 of these items are scored to give the general knowledge score, while 21 of the items are included for their discussion value
and do not enter into the score.

In the original validation and cross-validation of the SKAT, the reliability (KR-21) of the Knowledge Scale was found to be .87. The test-retest
reliability of this scale has not been determined. The validation sample of
851 medical students had a mean of 38.81 correst responses to the 50
scorable knowledge items ($SD = 5.78$).

Validity

There is evidence from a variety of sources to support the validity of the
Attitude and Knowledge Scales of the SKAT. All of the items in the
SKAT are straightforward and undisguised. Each question is intended to

obtain no more or less information than what is implicit in its meaning. Thus, the items in the SKAT are regarded as having *face validity*.

Evidence for the *construct validity* of the SKAT Attitude and Knowledge Scales comes from two general types of evidence: (1) correlations between the SKAT scales and selected items within the SKAT and (2) studies in which the SKAT was administered to subjects before and after some intervention expected to alter sexual attitudes and/or knowledge.

Table 1 presents evidence for construct validity based on an internal analysis of the interrelationship among SKAT items. These correlational data are based on a test sample of 850 medical students. The correlations in items 1 through 22 are product-moment correlations, while those in items 23 through 30 are point-biserial correlations. With an N of 850, correlations of .10 are significantly different from zero at the .01 probability level.

As can be seen in Table 1, each of the four Attitude Scales is related to other SKAT responses in a way that supports the meaning and interpretation of the scales. For example, liberal attitudes about heterosexual relationships (high HR scores) are associated with greater numbers of

TABLE 1

Correlations among the SKAT Scales and Selected Items from SKAT

Scale or Item and Response Number	Title or Item Content	SKAT-2 Attitudinal Scales and SKAT-2 Knowledge Scores					
		N	HR	SM	A	M	K
1. HR	Heterosexual relations	850		37	45	59	34
2. SM	Sexual myths	850	37		31	48	57
3. A	Abortion	850	45	31		45	32
4. M	Autoeroticism	850	59	48	45		49
5. K	Knowledge	850	34	57	32	49	
6. III(9)	Father's education	827	11	06	18	12	21
7. III(10)	Mother's education	840	11	10	14	15	18
8. IV(3)	Coital frequency	840	28	10	14	15	18
9. IV(4)	Variety coital technique	840	32	19	19	20	22
10. IV(5)	Variety coital partners	820	29	06	11	15	-02
11. IV(8)	No. of steadies	850	20	04	08	06	03
12. IV(9)	No. of coital partners	805	39	06	15	16	13
13. IV(10)	Rating, sexual experience	850	30	11	17	19	05
14. IV(11)	Rating, sexual knowledge	850	15	21	15	16	19
15. IV(13)	Home sexual permissiveness	850	-14	-07	-16	-07	-07
16. IV(14)	Conservative values	850	-48	-29	-27	-46	-41
17. IV(15)	Liberal values	850	36	18	25	27	31
18. IV(16)	Influenced by religion	850	-43	-21	-31	-35	-24
19. IV(17)	Value conflict with partners	850	23	10	10	18	13
20. IV(19)	Masturbation-Jr. High School	754	14	00	10	16	06
21. IV(20)	Masturbation-Sr. High School	754	14	04	11	23	19
22. IV(21)	Masturbation-College	754	10	07	07	21	15
23. III(2A)	Male	848	02	-20	00	-03	-08
24. III(3A)	White	832	00	12	10	13	21
25. III(7A)	Father-physician	843	12	07	08	20	11
26. III(7I)	Father-skilled manual	843	-15	-08	-20	-11	-05
27. III(11A)	Catholic	837	-11	02	-34	-13	-04
28. IV(22A)	Have used rhythm method	801	15	06	11	09	20
29. IV(24A)	Have used condom	803	24	05	16	09	23
30. IV(28A)	Have used pill	799	24	15	16	14	19

coital partners ($r = .39$) and a greater rejection of conservative social values ($r = -.48$). An increased tendency to reject sexual myths (high SM scores) is related to greater sexual knowledge ($r = .57$). Conservative attitudes about abortion (low A scores) are significantly associated with a Catholic religious preference ($r = .34$), and liberal attitudes toward masturbation (high M scores) are associated with greater frequencies of masturbation in senior high school ($r = .23$).

Evidence for the validity of the Knowledge Scale is more difficult to obtain from such an internal analysis of item inter-relationships, since it is less clear how one's knowledge about sexuality should relate to sexual values or behavior. It is noteworthy, however, that the highest correlation involving the Knowledge Scale in Table 1 is that between the Knowledge Scale and the SM Scale, the attitude scale which measures degree of acceptance or rejection of sexual myths. It would be expected, of course, that individuals who endorse or accept a wide variety of sexual myths would score lower on a test of sexual knowledge than those who are not accepting of such myths.

The second type of evidence for the construct validity of the SKAT scales—that obtained from SKAT testing before and after an intervention designed to change attitudes and/or knowledge—may be found in a number of published studies. For example, Marcotte et al[2] obtained pre- and posttest SKAT scores for a 1-week human sexuality course for first-year medical students and reported a significant increase on the Knowledge Scale and a significant change in the direction of greater liberalization of attitudes on all four Attitude Scales. Similarly, Mims, Brown, and Lubow[3] reported that a 5-day sexuality course resulted in significant increases on all the SKAT Attitude Scales except the Abortion Scale as well as a significant increase on the Knowledge Scale. Thus, support for the construct validity of the SKAT is provided by the fact that increases in sexual knowledge and liberalization of sexual attitudes, as measured by the SKAT, are shown to follow educational experiences designed to produce such changes.

USE OF SKAT

In view of the enormous number of people who have taken the SKAT, it is surprising that relatively little published research using the SKAT has appeared. This apparent paradox is most likely due to the fact that the SKAT has received its most widespread use in educational settings where it is used as a means of evaluating courses in human sexuality, not as part of controlled research. In those cases where educators have done research with the SKAT as an evaluation tool, it has typically been found to be a useful measure of the effectiveness of courses in human sexuality.[4-9]

One study found no significant changes in the SKAT after a course in human sexuality.[10] SKAT results have also proved useful in demonstrating the deficiencies of sexual health education.[11-18]

We believe that several additional research uses for the SKAT should be encouraged. First, although the SKAT would not be appropriate as the primary measure of outcome in sex therapy research, it would be of interest to determine whether the treatment of sex dysfunction affects the individual's sexual attitudes or knowledge. It would also be of interest to contrast the scores of individuals with and without sexual dysfunction on the SKAT scales. Finally, scores on the SKAT scales could be correlated with the sexual experience and personal background items of the SKAT[19,20] as well as with measures of sexual behavior, relationship variables, and individual personality variables.

REFERENCES

1. Lief H, Karlen A (Eds.): *Sex Education in Medicine*. New York, Spectrum, 1976.
2. Marcotte DB, Geyer PR, Kilpatrick DG, Smith AD: The effects of a spaced sex education course on medical students' sexual knowledge and attitudes. *Br J Med Educ 10*:117–121, 1976.
3. Mims F, Brown L, Lubow R: Human sexuality course evaluation. *Nursing Res 25*:187–191, 1976.
4. Chilgren RA, Rosenberg P, Garrard J: A process of attitude change in human sexuality. *J Med Educ 47*:779–784, 1972.
5. Garrard J, Vaitkus A, Chilgren RA: Evaluation of a course in human sexuality. *J Med Educ 47*:772–778, 1972.
6. Alzate H: A course in human sexuality in a Columbian medical school. *J Med Educ 49*:438–443, 1974.
7. Marcotte D, Kilpatrick D: Preliminary evaluation of a sex education course. *J Med Educ 49*:703–705, 1974.
8. Hadorn D, Grant I: Evaluation of a sex education workshop. *Br J Med Educ 10*:378–381, 1976.
9. Hoch Z, Kubat (Seidenros) H, Brandes JM: Results of the Sexual Knowledge and Attitude Test of medical students in Israel. In R Gemme, CC Wheeler (Eds), *Progress in Sexology*. New York, Plenum Press, pp. 467–482, 1977.
10. Golden JS, Liston EG: Medical sex education: The world of illusion and the practical realities. *J Med Educ 47*:761–771, 1972.
11. Kreger SM: Sexuality and disability. *ARN Journal* (Association of Rehabilitation Nurses) *2*:8–14, 1977.
12. Lief HI: Sexual knowledge, attitudes and behavior of medical students: Implications for medical practice. In Abse DW, Nash EM, Louden LMR (Eds.), *Education and Sexual Counseling in Medical Practice*. New York, Harper & Row, 1974.
13. Lief HI, Ebert RK: A survey of sex education in United States medical schools. In *World Health Organization Technical Report Series 572 (1975). Education and Treatment in Human Sexuality: The Training of Health Professionals*, 1975.
14. Ebert RK, Lief HI: Why sex education for medical students? In R Green (Ed), *Human Sexuality: A Health Practitioner's Text*, Baltimore, Williams & Wilkins, 1975.
15. Lief HI, Payne T: Sexuality: Knowledge and attitudes. *Am J Nurs 75*:2026–2029, 1975.
16. Lief HI: Sex education in medicine: Retrospect and prospect. In N Rosenzweig, F Pearsall (Eds), *Sex Education for the Health Professional*. New York, Grune & Stratton, 1978.
17. Elstein M, Gordon ADG, Buckingham MS: Sexual knowledge and attitudes of general practitioners in Wessex. *Br Med J 1*:369–371, 1977.
18. Elstein M, Dennis KJ, Buckingham MS: Sexual knowledge and attitudes of Southampton medical students. *Lancet*, 495–496, 1977.
19. Hoch Z, Kubat (Seidenros) H, Fisher M, Brandes JM: Background and sexual experience of Israeli medical students—National study. *Arch Sex Behav 7*:429–441, 1978.
20. Miller WR, Lief HI: Masturbatory attitudes, knowledge, and experience: Data from the Sex Knowledge and Attitude Test (SKAT). *Arch Sex Behav 5*:447–467, 1976.

Journal of Sex & Marital Therapy
Vol. 5, No. 3, Fall 1979

The Measurement of Marital Quality

Graham B. Spanier, PhD

ABSTRACT: The quality of marital relationships is the most studied topic pertaining to marriage and family life. Moreover, clinicians have become increasingly interested in this variable as divorce rates have climbed and as services for counseling and therapy have become more readily available and more widely accepted. These research and clinical needs necessitate the availability of measures of variables which assess marital quality (e.g., marital adjustment, satisfaction, and happiness). This article discusses the need for such measures, reviews the history of measurement in this area, identifies some conceptual and methodological issues of relevance, and then focuses most specifically on the Dyadic Adjustment Scale developed by Spanier. Some cautions for clinicians are noted, and a discussion of future measurement needs is presented.

The quality and stability of marital relationships has received much attention in modern social science. Marital quality, adjustment, success, stability, and satisfaction are the most frequently studied aspects of marriage and family relationships today. Lewis and Spanier[1] were able to identify more than 300 studies which examined some dimension of the quality of marital functioning. This interest is not surprising in light of the importance of marriage relationships in American society. Despite a record high divorce rate in the United States, marriage appears to be as highly valued as ever before; more than 9 out of every 10 Americans eventually marry, more than three-fourths of divorced persons remarry, and half of those who remarry following divorce wait no more than 3 years to form their new marriage.[2]

Clinicians as well as researchers have become increasingly interested in the quality and stability of marriage. With divorce rates high, counseling and therapy more widely available than ever before, and with a greater acceptance of mental health services among the population, persons in the helping professions have discovered a need to understand better the dynamics of marriage and family relationships. Moreover, they increas-

Dr. Spanier is Associate Professor of Human Development and Sociology, Division of Individual and Family Studies, The Pennsylvania State University, University Park, Pennsylvania 16802. Reprint requests should be sent to the author.

0092–623X/79/1500–0288$00.95

ingly desire to learn of instruments which might have value for diagnosis and treatment of marital dysfunction.

Both researchers and clinicians, then, are in need of carefully constructed instruments which can facilitate the study and/or treatment of marriage relationships. This article reviews the state of measurement related to the quality of marriage. The concept of marital quality is defined, measures of marital quality are reviewed, and the methodological issues involved in the design and use of such measures are considered. Special attention is given to the Spanier Dyadic Adjustment Scale.[3] Finally, issues of relevance to the clinician are presented, and some recommendations for future work in this area are made.

NEED FOR MEASURES OF MARITAL FUNCTIONING

In addition to the practical needs of professionals who study and treat marriages, there are other reasons why carefully constructed, well-tested measures of marital functioning are needed. Marriage is a complex phenomenon. Although it is possible to assess the quality of marriage by asking one or two global questions of the couple or one of the partners, such an approach often would not be sufficient to detect the complexity of the relationship, the range of potential or actual problems, or the special dysfunction which might pertain to the marriage in question. Thus, researchers have come to rely on specialized *scales*, which allow for a fuller examination of the many aspects of marriage.

For example, a single item such as "Everything considered, how happy would you say your marriage is? Is it . . . extremely happy, somewhat happy, somewhat unhappy, or extremely unhappy?" would give us a general indication of the overall quality of the marital relationship. However, it would not allow us to pinpoint problem areas such as religious differences, sexual dysfunction, in-law problems, or financial hardship. Consequently, there is general agreement that specialized study of marriage requires more sophisticated techniques which not only give a general indication of the state of the marriage, but also more specific information on particular problem areas. Moreover, some measures have subscales (e.g., the Spanier Scale[3]) which allow for an assessment of components of marital functioning, such as dyadic satisfaction, dyadic consensus, dyadic and affectional expression.

Since the first study of marital adjustment[4] 50 years ago researchers have recognized the need for scales that could tap the complexity of marriage. Scales have ranged from a few items to more than 100. Widely used scales today range from 9 items[5] to 32 items[3]. The most commonly used scale in the 1960s and early 1970s had 15 items.[6]

Scales that assess the quality of marriage have other uses as well. For example, they can be used to monitor changes in the institution of marriage itself through trend analyses of populations. The continuing development and refinement of such measures provides a barometer of changes in the variables which are most influential in marital functioning; as one component of marriage becomes less relevant over time, it should be less likely to be validated as an appropriate item for a measure of marital quality and thus would not be included in such a measure.

THE CONCEPT OF MARITAL QUALITY

A multitude of terms has been used by social scientists to reflect how well a marriage has functioned. At the most general level, there have been two basic types of assessment of marriage.[1] The first approach has been to focus on "marital stability," a term which refers to whether a marriage is dissolved by death or by divorce, separation, desertion, or annulment. A stable marriage is one terminated by the natural death of one spouse. An unstable marriage is one willfully terminated by one or both spouses. A second approach has focused on the "quality" of marital relationships while they are intact. This concept is most directly concerned with how the marriage functions during its existence and how the partners feel about and are influenced by such functioning. The concepts "marital adjustment," "marital satisfaction," "marital happiness," "marital integration," and others have been used to describe the quality of marriage relationships. The term "marital quality" has come into use as the general concept which encompasses the more specific meanings of the others.[1,3,7]

What most of these concepts share in common is attention to the qualitative dimensions of the marriage relationship. *Marital quality*, then, has been defined as a subjective evaluation of a married couple's relationship, with the range of evaluations constituting a continuum reflecting numerous characteristics of marital interaction and marital functioning.[1] A couple can be placed on a continuum ranging from high to low quality rather than being considered fixed in a discreet category of high or low quality. High marital quality is thought to be associated with good adjustment, adequate communication, a high level of marital happiness, and a high degree of satisfaction with the relationship.

Although marital quality is considered a most general term reflecting how well a marriage functions, there are no published measures of this concept. All researchers have chosen to attempt assessment of one of the more specific concepts which comprise marital quality. The Spanier Dyadic Adjustment Scale, presented in more detail below, focuses on marital and dyadic *adjustment* as perhaps the most general of the measurable indicators of marital quality. Satisfaction, cohesion, consensus, and affectional expression are considered to be components of overall adjustment.

OVERVIEW OF MEASURES OF MARITAL QUALITY

During the 50-year history of the study of the quality of marriage, there have been hundreds of studies using dozens of different measures. Of course, many of these measures were developed for use in only one

TABLE 1
Overview of Published Measures of Marital Adjustment and Related Concepts*

Developer	Name of Scale	Year Published	Reliability	Validity	Number of Questions	Number of Respondents
Adams	Marriage Adjustment Prediction Index	1960	NR[+]	Predictive, Concurrent, and Construct	743[++]	100
Bernard	Success in Marriage Instrument	1933	.96 - .97 Split half	Content, Concurrent, Construct	100	115 males 137 females
Bowerman	Bowerman Marriage Adjustment Scales	1957	.80 - .90 Reproducibility	Concurrent	67	102 couples
Buerkle & Badgley	Yale Marital Interaction Battery	1959	.90 Reproducibility	Concurrent	40	186 adjusted couples 36 unadjusted couples
Burgess & Cottrell	Burgess-Cottrell Marital Adjustment Form	1939	NR	Content, Concurrent, Predictive	130	526 couples
Hamilton	Marital Adjustment Test	1929	NR	Concurrent, Construct	13	104 couples
Inselberg	Marital Satisfaction Sentence Completion	1961	NR	Concurrent	13	29 wives 80 couples
Katz	Semantic Differential as applied to Marital Adjustment	1965	NR	Content, Construct	20	40 couples
Locke	Marital Adjustment Test	1951	NR	Concurrent	29	201 divorced couples 200 happy couples 127 others
Locke & Williamson	Marital Adjustment Test	1958	NR	Concurrent	20	171 males 178 females
Locke & Wallace	Short Marital Adjustment Test	1959	.90 Split half	Content, Concurrent	15	118 males 118 females
Manson & Lerner	Marriage Adjustment Inventory	1962	NR	Construct	157	120 males 117 females
Manson & Lerner	Marriage Adjustment Sentence Completion Survey	1962	NR	Content	100	120 males 117 females
Most	Rating of Marital Satisfaction and Friction	1960	NR	Concurrent, Construct	65	40 females
Nye & MacDougall	Nye-MacDougall Marital Adjustment Scale	1959	.86 - .97 Reproducibility	None	9	1300 females
Orden & Bradburn	Dimensions of Marriage Happiness	1968	NR	Content, Construct	18	781 males 957 females
Terman	Marital Happiness Index	1938	.60 H-W Correlation	Concurrent	90	792 couples

*Adapted from Spanier (1976), Straus (1969) and original sources. This summary does not include related measures of variables such as marital interaction (Farber, 1957), marital strain (Hurvitz, 1965), or marital communication (Navran, 1967); some scales based on modification of earlier scales (Burgess & Wallin, 1953; Karlsson, 1951); indirect measures (Kirkpatrick, 1937); single-item measures (Rollins & Feldman, 1970); multiple-item measures not intended for use as scales (Burr, 1970); and scales with minimal information available on both reliability and validity.

[+]NR = Not Reported

[++]Not all questions in this scale were considered measures of marital adjustment particular study, while others have seen much use over the years. Few measures, however, have undergone extensive development involving careful assessment of validity, reliability, and relevance. Such assessments, however, should be mandatory in modern social science since adequate techniques and an appropriate knowledge base for such study are available.

Table 1 summarizes the key published measures of marital adjustment and related concepts developed prior to 1970. The footnote to the table indicates the selective nature of the scales chosen for presentation. Although these generally were the most prominent scales available for the study of marriage, it is clear that few of them adequately demonstrate and report validity and reliability, nor do they have a clear conceptual plan behind the scale development.

The sample sizes used for validation are acceptable for most of the scales. However, in only a few cases is any form of reliability reported. And most of the assessments of validity are rather weak. Yet some of these scales continue to be used with little question. Apparently, there is a widespread belief that any scale which has been used in dozens of studies can be considered valid simply because of the fact that it has been used so widely. Those familiar with the historical development of the study of marriage know that many of our most central concepts have come to be defined by the measures of them—rather than the other way around.

METHODOLOGICAL ISSUES

In addition to the various conceptual problems noted earlier, the study of marital quality has a history of sometimes profound methodological issues. One criticism has been that the scales may measure conventionality as well as marital adjustment, thus confounding the measure.[7] There has also been the issue of whether a marital adjustment scale really measures the *adjustment of the marriage* or the *individual's adjustment to the marriage*. This issue is highlighted by the finding that husbands' and wives' marital adjustment scores correlate as low as .04 in one study of divorced couples and generally correlate about .60. If a measure of adjustment was a "true" assessment of the marriage, it might be assumed that the husband's and wife's scores would be nearly identical.

Undoubtedly, measures of marital adjustment have most often assessed an *individual's* judgment of the quality of the marital relationship. Although a given husband and wife would be expected to have evaluations which are consistent at a most general level, it would be reasonable to expect that perceptions, marital expectations, and tendencies toward certain response sets would vary from spouse to spouse, thus resulting in somewhat different evaluations. No measure has been developed yet which could be considered an evaluation of the marriage per se. Researchers have tried techniques like combining or averaging a husband's and wife's score, but this approach is really just an interpolation between two individual's perceptions—it is not a true marriage score.

Response sets are potentially troublesome for assessment of marital quality. This problem is especially likely since marriage tends to be a highly valued social institution, and thus married couples may want very much to communicate a favorable evaluation of the marriage to the researcher. Some research has shown that social desirability response sets may not be the extensive problem that some writers have indicated, but more research is needed on this question.[8] Although the promise of anonymity and/or confidentiality may encourage the honest reporting of marital adjustment, psychological response sets are undoubtedly present to some degree, with some individuals reporting better adjustment than exists in reality.

Another methodological concern has been that scales of "marital" adjustment and related concepts have been intended for use with married couples only, and such scales often assume rather traditional marriage relationships. With an increasing number of couples living together outside of marriage, there has developed a need for more general measures of "dyadic" adjustment which can be used for unmarried, as well as married, couples. The Dyadic Adjustment Scale, discussed below, was developed with this need in mind, and it is applicable for studies of married or unmarried couples.

THE DYADIC ADJUSTMENT SCALE*

Despite the conceptual and methodological problems noted above, and the many others cited by various writers,[9-12] I have taken the pragmatic position that as long as the concepts of marital quality, adjustment, satisfaction, happiness, and others are used, researchers ought to have available the best possible measures of these concepts. It can be assumed that these concepts will continue to be studied, and paper and pencil measurements of them will continue to be needed and used. These assumptions led to the development of the Dyadic Adjustment Scale.[3]

Five conditions guided the formation of a definition of adjustment to begin the scale development process:

1. It would be distinguishable from other concepts.
2. It could be operationalized. In other words, a measure could be de-

Part of this section is adopted from G.B. Spanier: Measuring Dyadic adjustment: New scales for assessing the quality of marriage and similar dyads. *J Marr Fam, 38*:15–28, 1976. Copyrighted 1976 by the National Council on Family Relations. Reprinted by permission.

veloped that follows from and is consistent with the definition proposed.

3. It would account for all criteria thought to be important in the conceptualization of adjustment.

4. It would not be so abstract that it could not be conceptualized clearly nor would it be so specific that it could not apply to a study of all marriages.

5. It could allow for investigation of any nonmarital dyad which is a primary relationship between unrelated adults who are living together.

Dyadic adjustment was then defined as a process, the outcome of which is determined by the degree of troublesome dyadic differences, interpersonal tensions and personal anxiety, dyadic satisfaction, dyadic cohesion, and consensus on matters of importance to dyadic functioning. As a part of the scale development project, a factor analysis sought to confirm the presence of these five components of dyadic adjustment. Three of these components were found to exist (dyadic consensus, dyadic cohesion, dyadic satisfaction), and one additional component was discovered (affectional expression). These four identified components comprise the total dyadic adjustment scale, and each is a separately identified subscale with reported reliability estimates.

The scale development project was a multistage process, accomplished as follows:

1. All items ever used in any scale measuring marital adjustment or a related concept were identified. This search produced a pool of approximately 300 items.

2. All duplicate items were then eliminated from the original pool of items, thus leaving for further analysis all items previously used at least once.

3. Three judges other than the principal investigator examined all items for content validity. Items were judged unacceptable and eliminated if a consensus existed that an item did not meet content validity criteria. Items had to be relevant for relationships in the 1970s and judged to be indicators of marital adjustment or a closely related concept, as defined by Spanier and Cole.[7] This preliminary screening of items was necessary to avoid presenting the respondent with too lengthy a questionnaire.

4. Approximately 200 remaining items were included in a questionnaire with a standard complement of social background variables. Among the questionnaire's 200 items were several new items that were developed to tap areas of adjustment which I thought had been ignored in previous measures. In addition, sets of items and scales previously used were expanded in order to make them more complete. Finally, to test the hypothesis that alternative wording in a

fixed-choice dyadic adjustment scale might produce different results and unpredictable response sets, approximately 25 items were included with alternative wording in the question and in the fixed-choice response categories.

5. The questionnaire was administered to a purposive sample of 218 married persons in central Pennsylvania. The sample consisted primarily of working and middle-class residents of the area who worked for one of four industrial or corporate firms which agreed to cooperate in the study.

6. Questionnaires were mailed to every person in Centre County, Pennsylvania, who obtained a divorce decree during the 12 months previous to the mailing. These respondents were asked to answer the relationship questions on the basis of the last month they spent with their spouses. We obtained 94 usable questionnaires from approximately 400 persons whom we were able to locate.

7. A small sample of never-married cohabiting couples was given the questionnaire to determine potential problems in question wording and applicability of the scale for nonmarital dyads. These data were not part of the scale construction analysis.

8. Frequency distributions were analyzed and all items with low variance and high skewness were eliminated.

9. Questions with alternative wording, structure, and category choices were further examined. Where differences in response variation were significant, items with the lesser variation were excluded.

10. Remaining variables were analyzed using a t-test for significance of difference between means of the married and divorced samples. Items that were not significantly different at the .001 level were eliminated. Following application of this stringent criterion, 52 variables remained.

11. Remaining questions with alternative wording were reexamined and items with the lowest t-value were excluded. At this point 40 items remained.

12. The remaining 40 variables were factor analyzed to assess the adequacy of our definition, determine the presence of hypothesized components, and make a final determination of items which were to be included in the scale. After 8 were eliminated due to low factor loadings (below .30), 32 items remained.

13. The issue of variable weighting was considered. After empirical comparisons were considered, using alternative weighting procedures and consideration of the scaling literature, a decision was made against weighting.

Evidence was provided for content, criterion-related (concurrent), and construct validity. The overall scale reliability was .96 for the final 32-item measure. Subscale reliabilities ranged from .73 to .94.

The Dyadic Adjustment Scale is designed to serve a number of different needs. First, for those wishing to use an overall measure of dyadic adjustment, the 32-item scale can be completed in just a few minutes, is only two pages in length, can easily be incorporated into a self-administered questionnaire, and can be adapted for use in interview studies. The scale, additionally, is useful since it allows researchers with more limited needs to use one of the subscales alone without losing confidence in the reliability or validity of the measure. For example, researchers interested specifically in dyadic satisfaction may use the 10-item subscale for this purpose. The format of the scale allows for easy coding or scoring. I have not been able to deal adequately with the problems of direction-of-wording and halo effects, but I have attempted to structure the scale in a way that encourages the respondent to think about each of the items being presented.

The scale has a theoretical range of 0–151. The source of the items included in the scale varies considerably. Some will be found in previous scales, others are modifications of items used previously, and others were developed specifically for the present study.

The scale is available in the appendix of the Spanier[3] article which reports on the development of the measure. More than 150 studies are currently using the scale. Since the measure was published relatively recently, there are only a small number of studies using the scale that already have been published. Additional research undoubtedly will begin to appear in the published literature with time. Until a larger body of published literature which uses the scale is available, it is recommended that researchers rely on the reliability estimates, means, standard deviations, and other descriptive information available from the original study on which the scale development was based.

USES AND CAUTIONS FOR THE CLINICIAN

All of the scales designed to measure marital quality appear to have been designed soley as research instruments. Such measures largely have been intended for group administration or for individual administration as part of sample surveys; they generally have not been intended for use in individual or couple diagnosis or treatment. Moreover, the methodologists who develop such scales historically have been reluctant to say that the measures should be used for clinical purposes. It has been customary for these researchers to caution against using marital quality measures for any other purpose than the assessment of group characteristics. Yet, it is reasonable to wonder why a well-developed scale of marital quality which meets stringent measurement criteria could not be used for clinical as well as research purposes.

The measurement of marital quality thus is in contrast with the measurement of other domains of social and psychological functioning. Many scales exist for diagnostic purposes related to individual psychological or emotional adjustment, even though it is well known that many of these measures suffer from some of the same as well as some different shortcomings found in measures of marital functioning. It can be argued that the methodologies appropriate for both the development of scales intended for diagnosis and scales intended for research are not different—or at least ought not to be when executed properly. General principles of scale development ought to apply for measures, regardless of the ultimate objectives. Only the methods of validity assessment might be given different emphasis; for example, predictive or concurrent validity might be especially important for measures used for clinical diagnosis, whereas content and construct validity might be sufficient for scales used only for research purposes.

Why have the designers of scales that assess marital quality shied away from recommending the use of their measures for individual assessment? One explanation is that the methodologist must accept greater professional responsibility by acknowledging that the scale may have direct relevance for individual decision making. The designer of the measure must be confident that the instrument will yield valid and reliable information about the individual or couple being assessed, if this information will be used to formulate a treatment plan or to guide otherwise decisions about the future of the relationship. This dilemma has been easy for marriage and family methodologists to avoid, since there has been little demand for measures to meet these individualized needs. But it is now reasonable to expect the development of measures with a degree of confidence in reliability and validity which would warrant their use in marital therapy. We are led, then, to a statement about the Dyadic Adjustment Scale.

The Dyadic Adjustment Scale has passed a good deal of scrutiny with regard to relevance, reliability, validity, and methodological rigor. As with other scales of its kind, it was originally intended for use as a research instrument and not for individual or couple diagnosis. However, it is my opinion that the scale can be used confidently in this way if it is used cautiously. The scale should not be used to make a judgment about whether a couple is happily or unhappily married, for example, on the basis of comparing their total adjustment scores with the norms presently available. First of all, there is too little published data on the scale to warrant such a conclusion at present. Second, one must be aware of the size of the standard deviations surrounding the mean scores for the married and divorced groups used to validate the scale. One may deviate substantially from the mean and still be considered within a "normal" range, depending on one's definition of normal.

The scale has no previously identified response or set of responses that can be used to discover those who might be considered especially maladjusted. Only norms may be used to give some indication of what is atypical, and as mentioned above, this is an imprecise undertaking. Finally, the items which comprise the scale each cover domains of marital functioning which are complex and which interact with the other domains. Thus, an individual item should be used cautiously as an indicator.

The scale could be used best in one of three ways: first, as a very general indicator, to help formulate an overall impression of the quality of the marital relationship; second, a husband's and wife's responses can be compared, and the similarities and differences used as a starting point for discussions; third, specific problem areas can be identified by examination of responses to individual items or to the subscales, and these responses can serve as a basis for discussion and for the development of a treatment program. It is recommended that the scale never be used alone for diagnostic purposes, without a complete interview and that it be considered a general guide and an auxillary tool in therapy. In this way the scale may have considerable value for the clinician.

FUTURE NEEDS FOR THE ASSESSMENT OF MARITAL FUNCTIONING

The Dyadic Adjustment Scale is a useful paper-and-pencil measure of marital quality. It is an improvement over earlier measures of its type, but it continues to have some of the same limitations inherent in all measures of marital adjustment and related concepts. Other measures of the quality of marital relationships will be needed for specialized purposes. Although the Dyadic Adjustment Scale seems to be a suitable measure for use in survey research studies and as a tool in clinical diagnosis, there are many other purposes for which other measures will be needed.

For example, measures that can be used in therapy for the more explicit diagnosis of problems influencing marital functioning are needed. Measures currently available can suggest problem areas, but marital interaction is complex, and current measures are not sensitive enough to uncover the dynamics of the problems which exist. Perhaps it is not likely that an instrument could be devised which, for example, could discover that the husband's impotence is heavily influenced by the wife's constant nagging about the husband's excessive spending of family income. A paper-and-pencil measure of marital adjustment might uncover that sexual relations, family finances, and perhaps communication were problems, but it certainly would not reveal the dynamics and complexities of such problems. It would be a tremendous step forward in marriage and family measurement if such interactional dynamics could be assessed better through measurement techniques.

Measures with more extensive attention to criterion-related validity are needed. Scales that are able to predict marital quality or to identify likely future problem areas also are needed. There were some early attempts to design such measures, but little work has been done recently in this area. Finally, measures are needed that can be used in laboratory and observational research and that can be used by individuals and couples without extensive professional supervision.

REFERENCES

1. Lewis, RA, Spanier GB: Theorizing about the quality and stability of marriage. In WR Burr, R Hill, FI Nye, IL Reiss (Eds), *Contemporary Theories about the Family.* New York, Free Press, 1979.
2. Glick PC, Norton A: *Number, Timing, and Duration of Marriages and Divorces in the United States: June, 1975.* Current Population Reports, Series P-20, No. 297. U.S. Bureau of the Census. Washington, DC, U.S. Government Printing Office, 1976
3. Spanier GB. Measuring dyadic adjustment: New scales for assessing the quality of marriage and similar dyads. *J Marr Fam 38*:15–28, 1976.
4. Hamilton G: *A Research in Marriage.* New York, Boni, 1929.
5. Nye FI, MacDougall E: The dependent variable in marital research. *Pacific Soc Rev 2*:67–70, 1959.
6. Locke HJ, Wallace KM: Short marital adjustment and prediction tests: Their reliability and validity. *Marr Fam Living 21*:251–255, 1959.
7. Spanier GB, Cole CL: Toward clarification and investigation of marital adjustment. *Int J Soc Fam 6*:121–146, 1976.
8. Dean DG, Lucas WL: Improving marital prediction: A model and a pilot study. Revised version of paper presented at the annual meeting of the National Council on Family Relations, St. Louis, October 1974.
9. Edmonds V, Withers G, Dibatista B: Adjustment, conservatism, and marital conventionalization. *J Marr Fam 34*:96–103, 1972.
10. Hicks M, Platt M: Marital happiness and stability: A review of the research in the 60's. *J Marr Fam 32*:553–574, 1970.
11. Laws JL: A feminist review of the marital adjustment literature: The rape of the Locke. *J Marr Fam 33*:483–516, 1971.
12. Lively E: Toward conceptual clarification: Case of marital interaction. *J Marr Fam 31*:108–114, 1969.

Table Citations

Adams CR: *Marital Happiness Prediction Inventory.* University Park, Pa., Division of Marriage and Family Service, 1960.
Bernard J: An instrument for measurement of success in marriage. *Am Soc Soc 27*:94–106, 1933.
Bowerman C: Adjustment in marriage: Overall and in specific areas. *Soc Soc Res 41*:257–263, 1957.
Buerkle JV, Badgley RF: Couple role-taking: Yale Marital Interaction Battery. *Marr Fam Living 21*:53–58, 1959.
Burgess EW, Cottrell L,Jr: *Predicting Success or Failure in Marriage.* Englewood Cliffs, NJ, Prentice Hall, 1939.
Burgess EW, Wallin P: *Engagement and Marriage.* Philadelphia, Lippincott, 1953.
Burr W: Satisfaction with various aspects of marriage over the life-cycle: A random middle-class sample. *J Marr Fam 32*:29–37, 1970.
Farber B: An index of marital integration. *Sociometry 20*:117–134, 1957.
Hamilton G: *A Research in Marriage.* New York, Boni, 1929.
Hurvitz N: The measure of marital strain. *Am J Soc 65*:610–615, 1965.
Inselburg RM: The sentence completion technique in the measure of marital satisfaction. *J Marr Fam 26*:339–341, 1964.
Karlsson G: *Adaptability and Communication in Marriage: A Swedish Predictive Study of Marital Satisfaction.* Uppsala, Sweden, Almqvist and Wiksells, 1951.
Katz M: Agreement on connotative meaning in marriage. *Fam Process 4*:64–74, 1965.

Kirkpatrick C: Community of interest and the measurement of marriage adjustment. *Family 18*:133–137, 1937.

Locke HJ: *Predicting Adjustment in Marriage: A Comparison of a Divorced and Happily Married Group.* New York, Holt, 1951.

Locke HJ, Wallace KM: Short marital adjustment and prediction tests: Their reliability and validity. *Marr Fam Living 21*:251–255, 1959.

Locke HJ, Williamson RC: Marital adjustment: A factor analysis study. *Am Soc Rev 23*:562–569, 1958.

Manson MP, Lerner A: The Marriage Adjustment Sentence Completion Survey Mannual. Beverly Hills, Calif, Western Psychological Services, 1962.

Most E: Measuring changes in marital satisfaction. *J Soc Work 9*:64–70, 1964.

Navran L: Communication and adjustment in marriage. *Fam Process 6*:173–184, 1967.

Orden S, Bradburn N: Dimensions of marriage happiness. *Am J Soc 73*:715–731, 1968.

Rollins B, Feldman H: Marital satisfaction over the family life cycle. *J Marr Fam 32*:20–27, 1970.

Spanier GB: Measuring dyadic adjustment: New scales for assessing the quality of marriage and similar dyads. *J Marr Fam 38*:15–28, 1976.

Straus MA: *Family Measurement Techniques* Mineapolis, University of Minnesota Press, 1969.

Terman L: *Psychological Factors in Marital Happiness.* New York, McGraw-Hill, 1938.

Journal of Sex & Marital Therapy
Vol. 5, No. 3, Fall 1979

Book Reviews

STEPHEN B. LEVINE, MD, EDITOR

MARRIAGE AND MARITAL THERAPIES, edited by T. J. Paolino, Jr., and B. S. McCrady. New York, Brunner/Mazel, 1978. 586 pages. $25.00.

Paolino and McCrady have furnished a useful reference for those interested in reflecting on their work with distressed marriages. Concepts which were previously widely dispersed throughout various mental health literatures are now conveniently consolidated in a single volume. Since few professionals are well versed in more than one mental health perspective, most readers will probably be unfamiliar with many of these ideas.

Marriage and Marital Therapies is excellent. It is exceptionally well conceived and can be profitably reread. It does not lend itself to being read in one or two sittings because of its length and occasional tedium. The major problem is that many of the volume's clearly articulated, germinal notions may be missed because of reader fatigue. It is, therefore, best approached in small doses.

The book's core consists of three units—both theoretical and practical chapters—on the psychoanalytic, behavioral, and systems theory approaches to marriage. The book begins with an overview of twentieth-century trends in marriage and ends with an erudite comparison of the three approaches. One chapter is devoted to a review of the research on the effectiveness of marital therapy. The entire book is more conceptual or intellectual than practical. Two of the chapters that were meant to be primarily practical focus a great deal on concepts.

The editors state their "firm conviction" in the preface that it is far better for

therapists to have some model of marriage than none at all. As each model is examined, however, it becomes clear that each leaves much to be desired. The models are often incompatible, making a grand synthesis of the perspectives impossible. Marriage, the arrangement that typically begins in young adulthood and is supposed to endure till the grave, contains so much complexity that there may be more danger than advantage in rigid adherence to a single model. Alan Gurman, in the concluding chapter, and the *tour-de-force* of the book, offers the following well-reasoned conclusion: "Therapists, as well as their patients, will fare better in the long run if they adopt an attitude of cautious optimism about the wisdom offered by current psychoanalytic, systems, and behavioral perspectives and accept none of them as a finished product." Gurman's chapter is vital to the book's balance. The authors of the core chapters, though cogent and persuasive, naturally emphasized the justifications of their perspectives—not the limitations. Gurman provides a critical, clinically sensitive, incisive examination of each perspective's advantages and limitations.

W.W. Meissner's exposition of a psychoanalytic perspective, while clinically rich, is somewhat limited and often tedious. Meissner's central hypothesis is that parental introjects, the basis of the child's sense of self, exert a lasting influence on the quality of future object relationships. Pathologic self-systems make marriage difficult because earlier parental conflicts interfere with the husband-wife relationship. Meissner's previous work on paranoid psychopathology provides the basis for much of this concept.

Most of the chapter is concerned with the origins of profoundly pathologic self-systems. The literature on family dynamics in schizophrenia is repeatedly discussed. More emphasis is placed on parent-child interactions than on the marital relationship. In fact, 15 pages of the introductory material precede the discussion of marriage! Among the issues notable for their absence are how to distinguish severe and mildly pathologic self-systems from those that are intact, conflicts and complexities inherent in adult relationships, how marriage may stabilize pathologic introjects and facilitate conflict resolution, and marital conflicts which stem from intrapsychic conflicts other than pathologic self-systems. Several subtle factors combine to detract from Meissner's presentation: a fatalistic use of the concept of psychic determinism; an assumption of superiority (e.g., "Psychoanalysis has at the minimum a headstart on the understanding of more complex social interactions"); a frequent disregard for precise definitions of terms (e.g., "The author has seen *any number* of cases in which the death of the significant figure in the grandparental generation will set up shock waves and reverberate throughout the whole of the family system and precipitate *pathologic reactivity* and *deviant expressions* in multiple members of the family system"). Nonetheless, there is much to consider in this chapter.

Carole Nadelson's chapter is an excellent theoretical and practical summary of a psychodynamic approach to marriage. Much of the material is a bit redundant, as it has been covered by Meissner. However, her perspective is broader, more balanced, and clearly based on work with couples. For example, "Marital conflicts occur because of differences in beliefs, interests, desires, values, expectations as well as from competition... differences in life stage or intrapsychic organization. Conflict is not necessarily destructive." My one criticism is that her remarks may mislead therapists into thinking that their formal brief evaluations should result in the same sophisticated grasp of the inter-personal system that she displays in this chapter. The following is a partial list of what she believes the initial evaluation should accomplish: a good developmental history; an understanding of each partner's coping ability, adaptational patterns, ego defenses (the differences between these three are not stated; neither does she mention how the task can be accomplished); self-image, how each partner manages affect, frustration, and disappointment; capacity for empathy, personal values, and goals of partners and their original families; why therapy was requested; the threat to the integrity of marriage; partners' conscious and unconscious motivations; why partners sought help when they did; marital identity. I do not believe Nadelson sufficiently stresses the fact that the evaluation of these and other factors is actually the essence of what the patient, and often the professional, calls treatment. The evaluation per se is merely an introduction to the real "evaluation."

Robert L. Weiss accurately described his chapter, "Marriage from a Behavior Perspective," by saying, "The odyssey has been long and touched many shorelines." His work is an honest, unpretentious, careful search for a perspective based on observation. Early in the chapter he tells the reader that behavior modification is not a theory of intimacy in committed relationships; rather, it is the technology derived from learning principles. A lengthy vocabulary list for these principles is provided. The concepts are illustrated by geometric figures that depict the interaction between significant variables. His view of behavior within relationships is quite dynamic or systems-oriented. He believes relationships function on a give-to-get principle in a sensitive changeable equilibrium. He develops a model of marriage in terms of four functions: objectification; support-understanding; problem solving; behavioral change. Unfortunately, almost one-third of the chapter is devoted to supporting this model with a literature review. Although the individual components of his review are well done, the entire chapter constitutes arduous reading. The chapter does provide a good picture of the highly specific behavioral sequences with which behavioralists are concerned.

K. Daniel O'Leary and Hillary Turkewitz provide a thorough description of the behavioral techniques employed with distressed couples. They begin their chapter with a vignette about the successful treatment of a specific couple with a combination of five techniques. Unfortunately, the couple is never mentioned again. The lengthy description of the four stages of treatment (courtship, engagement, marriage, disengagement [cute!]) which comprises the bulk of the chapter would probably have been more interesting as a chronicle of the couple's progress. The authors provide much discussion of how and when specific techniques are employed. The chapter provides an interesting contrast to Nadelson's. These authors are interested in specifying and correcting the dysfunctional behaviors—not in dwelling on such traditional things as the past, motivation, and transference. The avoidance of such complexities, the elementary nature of some of the recommendations (e.g., "Rapport can be facilitated by very careful, nonjudgmental listening to both clients"), and their incredible "possible" conclusion ("Interventions should be client-tailored to maximize effectiveness for a particular couple") contribute to a sense of oversimplification. The differences between psychoanalytic and behavioral conceptions of marital processes are quite apparent.

Peter Steinglass provides a careful, step-by-step conceptual development of systems theory. His chapter begins with a wonderful example of the same couple getting radically different sets of instructions from each of three prominent systems theory practitioners. He stresses the fact that systems theory, as applied to marriage, is more like a group of loosely connected concepts than an integrated theory. Yet he develops these concepts skillfully with a minimum of extraneous

detail. The long chapter soon gets ponderous as he highlights the dimensional differences between various versions of systems theory. This complexity requires careful study. In spite of Steinglass's repeated comments about its limitations, one has the sense that this theory is something profound, correct, and potentially quite revolutionary. This is particularly fascinating because basic notions such as the past and motivations are avoided.

Steinglass's chapter is followed by that of Carlos E. Sluzki—the most exciting in the book. The combined chapters make the unit on systems theory outstanding. Sluzki's relatively short chapter has significant conceptual, practical, and heuristic value. The prologue and conclusion are succinct but powerful. The bulk of the chapter consists of 18 prescriptions for therapeutic interventions—rules which are intended to illuminate the functions of symptoms in marital systems.

Neil Jacobson reviews the research on the effectiveness of marital therapy. The fact that there are no psychoanalytic or systems theory outcome data to review makes his task easier. He has only the burgeoning behavioral literature to organize, digest, and criticize. His very thorough, rigorous, but seemingly endless, critical review of published studies suggested to me that his exacting methodologic requirements can never be met and he basically does not understand why. His chapter should be read in conjunction with its critique in the final chapter by Gurman.

All things considered, *Marriage and Marital Therapy* is a fine book for both students and seasoned professionals. It provides a sobering update on attempts to assist couples with distressed relationships. It fosters no illusions about the ease of "fixing" marriages. As such, it is a welcome addition to the marital therapy literature.

Stephen B. Levine, MD
Case Western Reserve University

SEXUAL MORALITY: A CATHOLIC PERSPECTIVE, by Philip S. Keane, SS. New York, Paulist Press, 1977. 236 pages. $5.95.

Father Philip Keane is described on the book jacket as a noted professor and moral theologian at St. Mary's Seminary in Baltimore. This book carries a "Nihil Obstat" and "Imprimatur"—which means it has been officially declared free of doctrinal or moral error.

The book deals with sexual morality from a specifically Roman Catholic point of view. It is a "survey of moral perspectives on human sexuality," not a question-and-answer book. It begins with a theological overview of human sexuality and examines the role of women, particularly the feminist liberation movement. In these chapters Father Keane stresses that while human sexuality is basically good, there is a need for a moral perspective.

The second chapter deals with the elements of masculinity and femininity seen in both men and women. Chapter 3 is a description of the fundamental themes of Catholic moral theology. There are six main themes: (1) meaning of sin, (2) moral growth and moral development, (3) renewed understanding of natural law, (4) moral absolutes, (5) moral evil, (6) conscience and the Church's magisterium and discernment of spirit. These themes are discussed in terms of the traditional Roman Catholic approach and the evolution of moral thinking. The upshot of this chapter is that a good deal of responsibility is shifted to the individual and away from authoritative black-and-white prescriptions and permissions. This chapter stresses logical thought—but it may be a bit tedious.

Chapters 4 through 9 deal with specific issues of human sexuality: masturbation; homosexuality; heterosexual expression in marriage. The latter is the longest section in the book and is broken down into a consideration of specific sexual acts between partners, premarital and extramarital sexual activities, birth control and sterilization issues, divorce and remarriage. The remaining three chapters are devoted to sexuality and celibacy, including sections on rape, sexual dysfunctions, and therapy. The final topic is the recent Vatican document on sexual ethics.

The overall effect of the book is to give a considerably broadened point of view for the Roman Catholic individual. It basically affirms that sex and sexual expression are good and that human sexuality is God's gift. Father Keane cautions against an overpreoccupation with the physical aspect of sex. It is nice to see a reasoned discussion which concludes that procreation, however good, is not the only end of human sexuality.

This plea for a holistic vision of sexuality is echoed throughout the entire work. The liberalized sections on masturbation and homosexuality should help many individuals to feel more comfortable. The chapter on marriage emphasizes the richness that results when physical sexual pleasure is incorporated into a marital relationship. The question of the greatest good—rather than the lesser evil—is considered the end point in a discussion of the types of sexual stimulation used in marriage. An updated view of various contraceptive techniques is also presented—along with a reaffirmation of the traditional antiabortion stand. There is a discussion about when the soul is infused in relation to conception. It is implied that there is a 2-week period during which intervention is permissible, such as in a patient who has been raped. Subsections on divorce and remarriage reflect a contemporary approach.

The general tone and format of this book make it an extremely valuable volume for any practitioner of sexual therapy. I think many Roman Catholic patients would also find it helpful in defining their thinking about their own sexual practices. I found this book most useful in clarifying my own thinking about Roman Catholic stances. I highly recommend it to teachers of sexuality courses and to practitioners of sexual therapy.

Dennis H. Smith, MD
Case Western Reserve University

Journal of Sex & Marital Therapy
Vol. 5, No. 3, Fall, 1979

Audio/Visual Review

OLIVER J. W. BJORKSTEN, MD, EDITOR

EDCOA: OVERCOMING ERECTION PROBLEMS. Parts One and Two. Super-8mm sound, color cartridge (also 16mm and TV cassette). Source: Edcoa Production, 310 Cedar Lane, Teaneck, N.J. 07666. Cost: 1–5 films at $250.00 each, 6–8 films at $232.50 each, 12+ films at $215.00 each. 36-month lease (with $1.00 purchase option): 7 or more films at $8.90 per month. Special introductory purchase offer: 8 films at $250.00 each plus free Technicolor Series 2000 Movie Projector Viewer.

These films are the two most recent additions to the Edcoa sexual counseling film series and are intended to be used in conjunction with conjoint behavioral therapy of psychogenic erectile insufficiency. The film format is similar to that employed in the films on the treatment of premature ejaculation (*Stop and Go*) and consists of the clothed couple talking to an unseen therapist with flashbacks to the couple performing the behavioral exercises in their own bedroom.

Part One of the two-part series opens with Bonny and Bruce discussing the impact of the sexual difficulty on their relationship. He speaks of his previous period of intense frustration and discouragement, and Bonny discusses her guilt, anger, and loneliness. Later, Bruce states that he has learned that he cannot will an erection. He also discusses the role that performance anxiety and "spectatoring" played in his difficulty. The content of these discussions is good; however, the discussion is somewhat stilted and unconvincing. Bruce appears to be delivering a formal speech to an audience, and Bonny occasionally rolls her eyes as if trying to remember her next line. The flashbacks

consist of nongenital sensate focus, then genital sensate focus.

Part Two again opens with Bonny and Bruce in the therapist's office. Bruce talks about how he has learned that he does not have to have erections on every sexual opportunity and how "spectatoring" had inhibited his sexuality. Bonny discusses how she had unwittingly contributed to his difficulty. The discussion in Part Two is far more realistic and less stilted than in Part One. The flashbacks start with Bonny using the "tease technique" to stimulate Bruce. This section is especially good as Bruce starts the exercise with a flaccid penis, often appears to have only a partial erection, and occasionally loses his erection temporarily. The sequence evolves to penile insertion using the female superior position and nondemand thrusting. This section is especially good as Bruce again temporarily loses his erection. The flashback closes with Bruce bringing Bonny to orgasm manually.

Of the two parts to this sequence, Part Two is clearly superior to Part One. Part One appears redundant with the Edcoa sensate focus series. I would not recommend purchase of Part One to someone who possesses the sensate focus series. However, I would strongly recommend purchase of Part Two. This is an excellent film and clearly illustrates the main exercises in the treatment of impotence.

The Edcoa sexual counseling series now contains films on sensate focus, premature ejaculation, and erectile problems. It is becoming increasingly attractive as a complete package to employ with behaviorally oriented sex therapy. The series is strongly in need of good films on the treatment of female anorgasmia. If one intends to use these films in couples group therapy of mixed dysfunctions, there is one foreseeable difficulty. Bonny is the same actress in both the premature ejaculation and impotence films. However, her partners are different men although they have the same first name.

This might detract from the film's usefulness if one is treating conventional couples.

R. T. Segraves, MD, PhD
University of Chicago

SEX THERAPY TRAINING

FACULTY: Clifford J. Sager, M.D.
Merle Kroop, M.D.

This two year program meets one morning a week for three hours, at a cost of $1,200 per year. Curriculum includes anatomy and physiology of sex; the influence of immediate and remote factors on the etiology and treatment of sexual dysfunctions. The couples—client model of treatment will be taught, but experience will also be gained in working with individuals and groups. Participants will be expected to carry some cases and supervision will be provided. Prerequisite—a minimum of two years past graduate clinical experience, which includes working in family and couple therapy.* Interested applicants send resumes and two letters of recommendation to:

Harry Blumenfeld
JBG Educational Institute
120 West 57th Street
New York, N.Y. 10019

* MSW, Ph.D. in Psychology, MS in Nursing or M.D. (Psychiatry) required

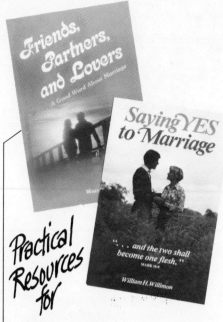